Get

STRONGER

By

STRETCHING

By

NOA SPECTOR - FLOCK

Body and movement are basic fundamentals just like our thoughts, senses, and feelings. Our physical body is the concrete aspect of our self; our muscular shape and tone are a mirror of our thoughts, feelings and patterns. In other words, we hold our attitudes in our body

Order this book online at www.trafford.com
or email orders@trafford.com

Most Trafford titles are also available at major online book retailers.

Whilst every effort has been made to ensure that the content of this book is as
technically accurate and as sound as possible, neither the author, the Hygienic Corporation, or the publishers can accept responsibility for any injury sustained as a
result of the use of this material.

Readers are advised to consult a doctor prior to beginning any exercise program.

Print information available on the last page.

ISBN: 978-1-5521-2368-3 (sc)

Trafford rev. 07/29/2019

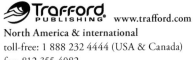 www.trafford.com

North America & international
toll-free: 1 888 232 4444 (USA & Canada)
fax: 812 355 4082

Acknowledgment

I would like to acknowledge the work of the following people who had patience with my English and contributed the time that was necessary to make this book come true. The Hygenic Corporation, the maker of the Thera-Band® products, which gave me the permission to use its product in my book; Don Musselman, who enriched my work with his wide knowledge of language, theater, and literature; My students who helped in the first stages of the creation:

Alexandra Hahl, who edited, organized, and helped put the manuscript into good form; Peter Hahl, who provided the illustrations; Angela Rauter, Marlow Fleming, Michael, and David who modeled for the exercises; to all my friends that were willing to read and give me their input and corrections, and to Geoffrey Arnold who did the last version photography.

Most important, each and every one of my students in school and workshops, clients, young and old, from whom I have learned what I now share. All of you have made this book possible, and I thank you.

Dedication

I was a bit nervous the first year that I taught at the University of South Florida in Tampa, Florida. My daughter Maya was about six months to a year old at the time, so I would bring her along with me as I taught my class, Movement Awareness in the Spirit of Feldenkrais. At that time, she was learning to roll, sit, crawl, and stand up. She showed my class exactly what I was trying to teach them about simple, efficient, developmental movement.

She actually did the teaching for me that year. It turned out to be one of my best years of teaching ever.

Thank you, Maya!

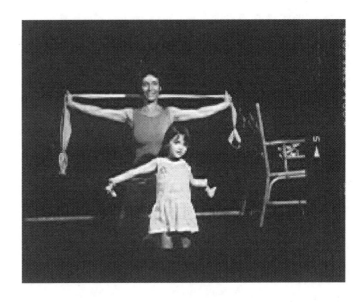

Preface

Dance and movement have been a major part of my life since childhood.

In Haifa, Israel at a young age, I would watch my mother teach yoga classes in our living room. It had large windows overlooking pine forests and the Mediterranean Sea. Mother would assemble her students teaching them with the belief that their improved physical health and well-being would come about by their practicing yoga breathing and exercise. These exercises were a combination of her astrological knowledge adapting to the changing seasons, months and conventional yoga.

At about 10 years of age, following my extended protests against the formal and stiff movement education I was subjected to in elementary school, I was provided with formal ballet lessons. I added self-expression at home, dancing freely to 78-RPM records of Tschaikovsky's "Sleeping Beauty" and "Sorcerers Apprentice".

These early experiences contributed to my sense of movement but I felt that both it and myself were lacking an inner core, a unifying force.

The centering I needed arose in an unexpected fashion. To arrive at dance class in downtown Haifa, I rode a city bus, which lumbered down the winding roads of Mount Carmel. Although the bus was equipped with leather straps for passengers to hold on to while it bounced over rough spots, I preferred to stand freely in the aisle and try to keep my balance. I wanted the challenge of adjusting my posture and alignment to adapt to the moving bus. When it would turn, accelerate or break to a halt, I would bend my knees, widen my stance, or breathe down into my pelvic floor.

My formal and self-studies were put on hold by compulsory two-year military service. At discharge, I was 20 and eager to return to dance training. I commenced studies with a professionally trained modern dancer, a practitioner of the Alexander technique. Her combination of skills aided me in developing a rich sense of space, diagonals and movement. In addition, I began to internalize the basic theories, principles and techniques of modern dance.

Yet I felt my movement was still imitative and not true to myself. I wanted to be authentic, for my dancing to arise out of universal truths and not the personality or philosophy of each teacher with whom I had studied. I needed a teacher to help me find these truths (as I had started to do by myself on the bus rides). To these I would develop and apply my unique expression. Ultimately, this led to my becoming the teacher I could not find.

During these searching periods, I studied the Feldenkrais method in Israel and in the United States. A method of re-education of the nervous system through movement awareness. For five years I was absorbed in this method, along with others, as I worked toward self-discovery. After I became a certified teacher of human movement and dance in 1981 in Tel Aviv, I was ready to incorporate my own knowledge of movement into other techniques of dance expression.

In 1982 I moved to Florida where I studied massage and other body techniques and modalities. I could now physically contact the body systems and have personal direct dialogue with them. In massage school, I was introduced to Thera-Band® but was dissatisfied with its narrow tube and the lack of support for the body part I was exercising.

But in 1990, while attending a workshop for teachers of dance, I again used the band, by now the wide version, which is easier to use. Once I held it, ideas flowed. I began to develop exercises using the band while as I worked with dancers at the Pinellas County Center for the Arts, St. Petersburg, Florida.

After eight years of teaching in Florida, I again felt the need to seek and search for greater depth. In 1991, I came across a wonderful guide named Bonnie Bainbridge Cohen- a teacher so intuitive and so profound that she evoked in me the process of inquiring and of learning to make distinctions among people's thinking, actions, and movements.

I hope to transfer some of the experience I have gained to you, the reader, as I share with you a safe and healthy technique of strengthening and stretching muscles with the aid of an elastic device called Thera-Band ®.

Table of Contents

Introduction

The focus of this book is an exercise program, which will teach you how to contract a specific muscle while lengthening it. This "eccentric contraction" (as explained later) will integrate the movement of a certain muscle with the surrounding joints and muscles in that area, in order to involve the whole body and to create harmonious movement.

The contraction occurs while lengthening and stretching the fibers, yet the number of participating fibers are deceases. Having less fiber share the load increases the tension. Consequently, the overload stress and tension creates greater stretch on the working fibers, resulting in enhanced flexibility. Michael J Alter in his book Science of Stretching writes about few studies relating to eccentric contraction. On page 80 "recently several studies actually published photographs showing some mechanical disruption of the z-lines. Their findings indicated that the z - lines during overloading constitute a potential weak link in the myofibrillar contractile chain. However, they noted that the structural disturbance may also be secondary, resulting from an activation of lysosomal enzyme, bringing about a concomitant inflation. Other researchers such as Abraham (1977, 1979) and Tullson and Amstrong (1968, 1981) also provide additional support for the relationship between muscle soreness and connective tissue irritation or damage.

This program will introduce you to Thera-Band ®*, an elastic device that can prepare you for any athletic activity. Using the band during your warm-up will simultaneously provide you with increased strength, flexibility, and circulation; it will improve your sensory motor skills, enhancing coordination and kinesthetic awareness. The exercises will help you learn how to initiate movement from the larger and stronger muscles within the center of the body (core). That creates efficient movement, and let the movement continue through to the smaller muscles in the extremities. This order will result in more efficient and more delicate movement for expression.

*(Friden, Sjostrom, and Ekblom, 1981; Friden, 1984; Newham, McPhil, Mills & Edwards, 1983; Newham, Mills, Quigley, & Edwards, 1983)

If you wish to order another Thera-Band® from the author Call 1-727- 345-2570 Email. noanik8@att.net
Hygenic Corporation can be reached: Tel 1-800-537-5512 [(216) 633-8460 Ohio residents], by fax (216) 633-8460, or by writing 1245 Home Avenue, Akron, Ohio 44310.

This book is divided into two chapters. Chapter 1 explains whole body movement. It contains discussions on stretching and strengthening, body alignment, and breathing. Chapter 2 is divided into muscle groups and areas, which will gain additional length and strength through proper attention and exercise using the body as a whole system.

The exercises will start from an easy level and build to a more difficult level by changing position of the body or by increasing the complexity of the exercise. You will be able to some in your bed; on the rug; on a chair, or standing up.

What is Tera-Band®?

Thera-Band®is an elastic band used in exercising for improving strength and range of motion, in addition to cooperation of muscle groups when used with out isolation. It is part of a whole group called resistive exercises. The band support and challenge the body as it stretches and returns to neutral.

The bands are available in latex and in latex free. They are similar in strength, but vary in width. 6" and 4" for latex free. You choose one of five 6" by 6' rubber bands of differing resistance levels to provide the tension.

% Elongation	50%	100%	150%
Red	2.5	4	5
Green	3	5	6.5
Blue	4.5	7	9
Black	6.5	9.5	12.5
Silver	8.5	13	17

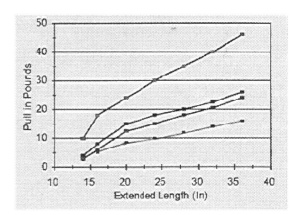

Getting Acquainted with Thera -Band®

First, examine the band. Hold it in your hands. Does it lay comfortably in your hand? How is the feel? What color is it? How thick is it? How wide? Sense its texture, softness and smoothness. Note the "chocolate smell" that rises from it. Take time to play with it. Do you have any sense to how much resistance this band exerts? The resistance increases as the band stretches and decreases as the band shortens back to its original position. Now stand and hold the band with both hands.

Experiment with the idea of isolating your arms from your torso. Next, involve the torso with the movements of your arms. Combine arm movement and torso moving. Now you are using more of yourself—the muscles of your torso and the muscles of your arms. You are thereby creating more flow. You are moving with integrated movement that will appear graceful. Next pay attention to your breath and with no special effort continue breathing through out the movement.

Care of the Band

The exercises in this book do not require any additional apparatus.

A simple double knots is sufficient The Hygienic Corporation, which produces the Thera Band®), also produces a set of handles, and Door Anchors to secure the end of the band. The handles can be attached to each end of the band. These can be used as an alternative to the band "loops" for some of the arm exercises, if desired. .

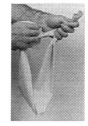

It is not recommenced to close the door on the end of the band; this leads to early tearing of the band. The band can be damaged by extreme heat or sunlight. It should be stored back into package or in a dark place, such as a drawer after each use. To keep the band soft and supple, sprinkle it with talcum powder or cornstarch.

Frequent questions –

Why Thera -Band®?

The Thera - Band is the only resistive band indorsed by the American Physical Therapy Association. More over it has developed and adapted by the sport industry later I have developed it as a tool for dancers, and now this book which is geared to the persons who are 50 years and older. It has been tested, tried, used and proven to be a good and effective product for conditioning, rehabilitation, and strength building. Research and study are at the base principles of the Hiegenic Company. The resistive bands have been clinically proven over 15 years to improve strength, range of motion, balance, functional activities. For more info please visit the Thera-Band® Academy on the net

Where to buy a band? –

A- Many resistance bands on the market are either too short or come in a package of few band which you do not need. For this program Get Stronger By Stretching you need a 6" wide and 6' long band.

The Hiegenic corporation web site is www.tera-band.com You may contact them to find a dealer close to you.

From the author - you may purchase a band from Noa Spector- Flock directly noanik8@att.net.

Or 1-727-345-2570

Through the Internet - Fitness Wholesale www.fwonline.com/tbands.htm

Out of the U.S.A.

Tel: 330-633-8460

Fax: 330 633-9359

Germany

Tel: 49-6433-91640

Fax + 49-6433-9164

What are the bands and tubing made of?

A. Thera-Band® resistive bands and tubing are made of natural rubber latex made into sheets and tubing. Latex-free Thera-Band® resistive bands are made of synthetic rubber. The trademarked colors indicate the resistance levels.

What forces are produced by the bands and tubing?

A. The force produced by bands and tubing is directly related to elongation. Each color will provide a specific amount of resistance at the same percent elongation, regardless of initial resting length. For example a 1-foot piece stretched to 2-feet (100% elongation) will have the same force as a 2-foot piece of the same color stretched to 4-feet. The force slowly increases as the band or tube is stretched.

Are there any specific conditions under which bands would be preferred over tubing or vice versa?

A. Typically, the use of bands or tubing is a matter of personal preference. Both bands and tubing demonstrate similar properties in progressive resistance. However, bands allow more surface area to be covered during some resistive exercises. In Get Stronger By Stretching we use the band.

How do bands and tubing compare to free weights (such as dumbbells)?

Elastic resistance has different properties than free weights, in that elastic resistance doesn't rely on gravity to produce force. Therefore, multiple patterns, speeds, and motions can be exercised with elastic resistance. Since the resistance increases with elongation, bands and tubing cannot be labeled with an absolute resistance level (e.g., yellow = 1 pound).

Do elastic bands and tubing provide similar results compared to free-weights?

A. Yes. Elastic resistance has been proven to be as effective as free weights in developing strength. Elastic bands and tubing are often substituted for free-weight exercises.

Doesn't the force increase at the end range, not allowing me to complete a full range of motion?

A. As with any resistive exercise, elastic resistance must be used properly. While the force of the bands and tubing does increase with elongation, the "strength curve" of elastic resistance is physiologically similar to human joint strength curves. This provides less torque at the beginning and end ranges, where the muscles can't produce as much torque.

How many repetitions will the bands or tubing withstand?

A. Elastic bands and tubing can last for a very long time with proper care and use. Thera-Band® elastic bands and tubing have been tested at over 10,000 repetitions without any breakage.

How long can I stretch the bands or tubing?

A. We don't recommend stretching beyond 300% elongation. The bands and tubing are more susceptible to breaking with greater than 500% elongation (for example, stretching a 1 foot piece to 6 feet), and the resistance increases sharply after 500%.

Why do the bands or tubing break, and what precautions should I take?

A. With normal daily use, the exercisers should last for many months. However, they won't last forever. They may break if stretched beyond 500% or if they are used with small tears or abrasions. These small tears and abrasions usually occur at the "connection point" of the band or tubing to an attachment device. Therefore, always inspect the band or tubing (particularly near the connection) before use. It is recommended to use the Thera-Band® Door Anchor, Exercise Handle, and Assist for connection. Be aware that jewelry, fingernails, and other sharp objects may cause small tears or abrasions. Always protect the eyes during exercise with elastic bands or tubing.

When should I replace my bands or tubing?

A. Always inspect your bands or tubing for signs of wear, including small tears, abrasions, or cracks before use. Pay particular attention to the connection point. Always replace the bands or tubing with any sign of wear. With heavy use, such as in a physical therapy clinic, bands and tubing should be replaced every 1-2 month. The bands and tubing will not last forever, and will experience normal wear and tear with extended use. However, they should be safe to use as long as there are no visible signs of wear

Can they be used in a chlorine pool?

A. Yes, but the product will deteriorate at a quicker rate due to the chlorine. After each use in the pool, rinse the bands in tap water and hang them to dry. For extended use on land, apply a light dusting of cornstarch before use.

Why and under what circumstances is it better to prescribe latex-free Thera-Band® bands over standard latex Thera-Band® bands?

A. The regular Thera-Band® resistive bands and tubing contain natural rubber latex. Latex allergies occur in a small percentage of the population (about 5-10%). When patients indicate latex allergy or sensitivity, they should use the latex-free bands. Also, patients with spina bifida tend to be more at-risk for latex allergy. Anyone using the latex bands or tubing that experience an allergic reaction (such as redness or swelling on the skin near the band) should use the latex-free bands.

How do the Thera-Band® latex-free bands compare with the original latex bands?

A. The resistance of latex and latex-free bands are similar.

Can Thera-Band® bands be purchased powder free?

A. The powder is used to keep the product from sticking to itself during manufacturing. The powder will
be removed with normal use, and is not necessary for proper functioning of the product. Thera-Band® Latex-Free bands, however, do not contain powder.

What is the shelf life of Thera-Band® bands and tubing?

A. When kept in a cool, dark environment, the bands and tubing should last for many years. However, use, exposure to temperature extremes, chlorine, and sunlight decrease the "shelf-life".

How do I connect the bands or tubing for exercise?

A. The Thera-Band® Door Anchor should be used to secure one end of the bands or tubing for exercise. It isn't advisable to tie the exerciser to a doorknob or to "close" them in a door; this leads to early breaking. The Thera-Band® Exercise Handles and Assist can be used to grasp the exercisers. To connect to the legs or arms, use the Thera-Band® Extremity Strap.

How does Thera-Band® brand compare to other brands?
A. The resistance values and color progression for Thera-Band® bands and tubing are specific to the brand, and cannot be applied to other brands.

What will you find in this book?

You will find some exercises that deal with different muscle groups in the body. These exercises are not just for strengthening or stretching them alone, but are a combination of both elements. The process you will learn (mentioned in the introduction) is called the "eccentric contraction," which will lengthen the muscle as you work it, thus making it stronger.

My main purpose in this book is to give you, the reader, an understanding of how to develop an "intelligent" body through proper breathing, posture, and the right exercise attitude. I hope to achieve this by emphasizing where to initiate the movement from, and how to develop the exercise into an efficient movement that uses the correct muscles with the right amount of tension in them.

Starting a Workout

If you are a beginner or a person who would like to get back into shape again, I would suggest that you follow the whole body program for a while (appendix D). Start with few repetitions, tow for example and build you strength and endurance slowly. If you are a professional dancer or athlete who exercises with the band, you may choose to concentrate on a specific area of the body one day (the upper body, for example), employing the appropriate exercises for it, and then concentrate on a different area the next day (like the lower body). This will rest the muscle groups and you will not overwork anyone area of the body. When you feel that your body "knows" the exercises—that is, when you feel strong enough for 12-15 repetitions and are fluent in your movement—then you may try another combination. Once you work with the book and fully understand its intent, then you may build your own program according to your creativity and needs.

You may use the exercises in this book as a means of warming up for other activities, taking into account that you "create space." Use your breath at all times, and move in the directions the body is designed to move in. Do not push against joints, tendons, or ligaments.

1. Read through each exercise, noting the photographs. The exercises are generally explained only to one side so you may learn how to do them; it is expected that you will also repeat them to

the other side. (NOTE: I have chosen Hebrew names for some of the exercises, followed by their translations. Also, the abbreviations "R" and "L" are used in place of "right" and "left," respectively.)

2. Once you understand the exercise, do it once on the specified side to get the basic feel of it, and then repeat it to the opposite side so your body will be worked equally on both sides.

3. As you get stronger, gradually increase the number of repetitions you do until you reach 12-15 times on each side. This way, you can build up muscle endurance—the ability of the muscles to sustain work over time and through the repetition of effort. Using 60-80% of your total muscle power will be sufficient to increase your strength.

The band will offer the resistance you need to gain both strength and endurance. In fact, an endurance baseline may be established by doing just 6-8 repetitions of each exercise regularly.

You can gauge the amount of resistance you are using and the rate of your improvement by the distance of the band stretch. The shorter the band, the greater the resistance will be (you may mark the band with a pen). (Refer to the color code and chart mentioned in the Introduction.)

When you design your program, make sure you keep in mind the needs of your particular sport or specialty. (For example, runners would have no need to concentrate on the outward rotation of the hip, to the degree ballet dancers would.)

Three sample workouts, located at the end of the book, are provided for you to use as a model for how to design your own individual workout routine. The sample workouts are a general three-part whole body program, and two specific programs for dance conditioning and swim conditioning, respectively.

Things to Remember

As a rule of thumb, consult your doctor for questions and complete physical before starting this or any new fitness program

You can gain the most from this book if you follow a few basic approaches:

1. *WORK SLOWLY.*

This means very slowly for two reasons:

A. The slower you work, the more control you will have over the movement.

B. By slowing down you can pay closer attention and learn "how" to do the exercises. You will learn which patterns you are already moving in. Once you know this, you will be able to change old patterns and relearn new ones.

2.   *USE YOUR BREATHING*

Keep the breathing rhythmic and constant. As a general rule, movements are the most efficient if they are executed while you are breathing evenly and continuously. There are methods that instruct a precise time for inhaling and exhaling for specific results. Here the objective is to breath continuously. Many times we find ourselves holding our breath on the effort of a movement. However, any movement will be easier to do if you conscientiously exhale as the effort is being carried out.

For example, if you are sitting on the floor with your legs straight in front of you, lowering your torso behind you toward the floor by using your abdominal muscles, you will fully exhale during the downward process. While down, pause to inhale, then again, fully exhale as you resume a sitting position. In other words, you should exhale on both the flexion and the extension (exertion and the return) of the movement.

3.   *PAY ATTENTION.*

Become aware of what you are doing so it will not become a mechanical movement. Establish the intention to make the connection between body and mind. The holistic approach (body, mind, and spirit) will bring better and faster results to your physical appearance and well-being. Always be aware of how the process is taking place and the parts of the body that are involved. (For example: by retracting the abdominal muscles you are able to raise your leg higher.)

4.   *MAINTAIN BODY ALIGNMENT.*

A.   When bending your knees, whether you are sitting, standing or lying down, you must create a straight, imaginary line that runs from the hip to the center of the knees, then to a point between the second and third toe. This will assure that you are developing all sides of your leg equally and not using one muscle over the others, which will prevent stress.

B.   While in sitting position, position yourself on top of your "sitting bones" (your ischial tuberosities) not in front, nor behind. Stack your vertebrae above it to create a balance where the bones, rather than merely your back muscles, will support you.

C.   When inhaling, or when lifting arms over your head, keep the rib cage tucked in. Imagine it to be like a closed umbrella rather than an open one. This will avoid unnecessary stress on the vertebra in your mid-back.

D.   Keep your head as a continuation of the back. Do not let the chin protrude forward; rather, bring it downward slightly and toward the spine.

E.   Keep 180 ° between the shoulders. Work on your balance between forward and backward (anterior and posterior).

F.   Never lock your knees or elbows. When you lengthen your legs, think of lengthening them from the back of the leg while pulling your heels out away from you.

5.   *MAINTAIN BODY POSITION.*

Pay attention to the position described for each of the exercises, which follow for best results.(For example, while exercising the abdominal area, it is important to maintain the arms in the specified position to work the latissimus dorsi.

6.   *WORK SIMPLY.*

Do not try to look nice by adding unnecessary gestures to the movement. Pay attention to how you use your body for the movement. Know the origin of the movement and how it is developed through the body to other parts. This will create a fully developed sequence which will be both efficient and in harmony with body movement.

7.   *WORK DEEPLY.*

Do not move only your extremities to "get some exercise." Rather, you should pay attention to your inner sensations. Move using the big muscles in the center of your body to initiate the movement; then make space in the joints to move the extremities.

8.   *CREATE SPACE.*

Throughout the book, the expression "making space in the joint" is used. This means, when you start to move a limb, do not push it into the joint in order to move it; instead, try to do the opposite: create the sensation of lengthening it out of the joint before even contracting the muscle to move. One good way to achieve this is to exhale while create the lengthening sensation. This is a safe way to exercise and will not irritate arthritic conditions. (For example, when lifting your arm above your head, think of the arm being pulled out from the shoulder joint before you lift it.)

9.   *WORK EVENLY.*

Remember we move in habitual patterns. Our bodies are not symmetrical and, therefore, are not symmetrically strong, long, or flexible. Pay attention to this, and work as evenly as possible to create new patterns. In this way, the load of the work can be shared more equally on the muscles, ligaments, tendons, and joints in the body.

10.   *BE AWARE OF YOUR RESISTANCE LEVEL.*

The shorter the distance is from where your hands are placed to the ends of the band, the more resistance you will have; doubling the band will double the resistance. You may also decide to move ahead to a stronger band when necessary, in order to increase your level of resistance.

Conclusion

I have constructed the exercises so they reach and work the muscles from different angles. For example, consider an exercise that flexes and extend of the thigh and knee. The advanced version would be to rotate the leg out while repeating the same exercise, which would affect additional (or entirely different) fibers of the muscle than doing it in the original position.

My main goal is to create strength and length in your body equally, so that both qualities will support and balance each other. More than that, my vision is that your body will then integrate efficiency and harmony of movement. This is why I chose exercises involving muscle groups and integrating areas. I hope that by following the instructions described, you will learn how to initiate movement from a strong muscle in the center of your body (for example—psoas), and to include more muscles as the movement develops and expands.

This way you can experience the full sensation of integrated whole body movement. Enjoy.

Noa Spector- Flock

WARNINGS:

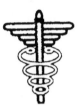

1. Use the exercises in this book with caution. Consult your doctor if you have any questions. Have a complete physical checkup before starting this or any new fitness program, especially if you have medical conditions such as: high blood pressure, varicose veins, bursitis or arthritis.

2. Use caution; Use your comfort as a guide, exercising the knees, lower back, and shoulder joints.

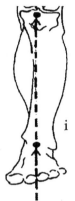

A. KNEE: The knee must be aligned with the second toe in all of the exercises to avoid eversion/inversion (twisting of the foot) that creates overload and strain. If you have an injury to your knee, you may avoid undue pressure by tying the band above the knee instead of below it. When doing leg exercises with such movements as abduction (bringing a body part away from the center line of the body), adduction (bringing a body part closer to the center line of the body) and turn in/turn out. Always bend your knees very slightly as you exercise to prevent hyperextension, especially if you have experienced this problem in the past.

B. LOWER BACK: For exercises done while lying supine (laying on the spine) on the floor, you should NEVER release the lower back in an arch greater than your normal posture. Holding and supporting the abdominal muscles against the lower back will keep the lower back from arching; exhaling on the effort will also help. The Transversus abdominis muscles will be engaged and contracted against the back, and all around creating a hollow sensation and look to the abdominal area (to distinguish from pelvic tilt). When in a standing position, allow the lower back to drop down with a very small pelvic tilt (hardly noticeable, mostly felt) to the front, so the spine is kept as straight as possible. Your knee position will also affect the lumbar area, so again, bend your knees slightly.

C. SHOULDER JOINTS: People with restrictions in their shoulder joints will have to use less resistance and increase the slack in the band. To improve, do only a very small portion of each movement. Try to isolate the feeling of lengthening the arm outward to "create space" in the joint before you actually lift it. You should also learn to use the muscles of the back to support the arms so that most of the effort will fall upon the bigger muscles (trapezius, latissimus dorsi, and the rhomboids), which are better suited for that function.

3. Keep the band away from young children and pets.

4. Cover sensitive areas of your skin or hairy areas of your body to prevent pinching or pulling.

5.   Secure long hair on top of the head.

6.   Keep the wrists straight to create a continuous line from forearm to and.

7.   Always pull the band away from body, be aware not to hit your face.

8.   Always be in control, while pulling and on the release to starting position.

9.   Check the band for possible damage before use.

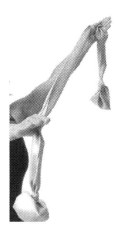
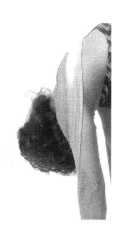

Chapter 1

ACHIEVING WHOLE BODY MOVEMENT

Organic learning is essential. It can also be a therapeutic in essence. It is healthier to learn than to be a patient or even be cured. Life is a process not a thing. And, processes go well if there are many ways to influence them. We need more ways to do what we want than the one we know - even if it is a good one in itself.

-- Moshe Feldenkrais.
The Elusuve Obvius (1981:29)

STRETCHING AND STRENGTHENING

If you ever been back stage, or even in a dance studio, you probably saw dancers as they are constantly stretching their muscles to increase their flexibility and their range of motion, especially in the hip socket, spine, and feet. However, strength is the other side of flexibility. Too much flexibility in the muscles without adequate strength will result in uncontrolled mobility, loose joints, and overall weakness. This condition will too often result in injury. On the other hand, too much strength without much flexibility will limit the range of motion. For a muscle to become stronger one needs to increase the period of time, the frequency and the intensity; that in this case is by using the band. For the muscle to become more flexible, it must be stretched for a specific length of time.

The ideal situation would be to create a balance between the two elements, which will provide many benefits:

1. The range of motion (ROM) will be increased, and it will continue to evolve as the strength in the body also increases. In other words, we will assume that you can stretch your leg beside you to a certain point. It is only after you acquire the strength to hold it there that you can work on stretching your leg higher. Flexibility is great only if you have the strength to use what you have while you are moving.

2. A combination of exercises that both stretches and strengthens the muscles will promote a better blood supply (and therefore, a better oxygen supply) to the muscles and the organs. This means a better workout on the day you exercise and less soreness on "the morning after."

3. As we stretch the muscles, we will also elongate the fascia, which supports and holds the muscle fibers together, and connects the muscle groups.

4. By strengthening a muscle at the same time we keep it long and flexible, we will prevent injuries around the joint, such as ligament sprains, tendon strains, and joint subluxation.

Definition of Terms

Types of Muscle Movement

Muscles can be contracted, relaxed or elongated. This happens on a chemical level as well as on a physical level. The changes in the muscle length are due to the thick and thin myofilament (actin and myosin) sliding along each other.

A CONTRACTION builds tension in the muscle fibers, generates movement, functions in posture maintenance, and produces body heat. Chemically, a contraction occurs when calcium is released into the muscle body.

The place where the nerve and the muscle meet is called neuromuscular junction. When an electrical signal crosses that junction it is transmitted deep inside the muscle fibers. In the muscle fibers, the signal stimulates the flow of calcium. The thick and thin myofibrils are now sliding across one another. This action causes the sarcomer to shorten, which generates force. In the muscle there are billions of sarcomeres. They obey the law of 'all or none' and when a fiber contracts it contracts completely. Not all of the fiber of a given muscle needs to contract at the same time. The more force needed, the more fibers will be recruited to the job. The mitochondria is the part of the cell that converts glucose into energy. There are different types of muscle fiber with different amounts of mitochondria. These fibers are categorized as slow twitching and fast twitching. The slow ones are slower to contract but also slower to fatigue. The fast ones are very quick to contract and come in two types: type 2A fatigues at an intermediate rate; type 2B fatigues very quickly. They are present in a given muscle in varying amounts and will be recruited, initially type 1, then type 2A, and, if needed, type 2B. Relaxation is totally passive. When the muscle fibers no longer receive impulses, they let go, they relax. In other words, there is no more generation of muscle tension because the calcium that was there has withdrawn.)

RELAXATION is totally passive. When the muscle fibers receive no more impulses, they let go; they relax. In other words, there is no more generation of muscle tension because the calcium that was there has withdrawn.

STRETCHING can occur when a force outside a particular muscle is used. This force can be 1. gravity, 2) body motion, 3) an antagonist muscle working in opposition to the muscle being activated (hamstring versus quadriceps), or 4) another person or machine pulling on the body part. With the band, we mostly contract eccentrically, meaning we will build tension while elongating the muscle. The stretching combined with the resistance of the band makes the muscle stronger. For eccentric contraction to occur the entire muscle group must work its full range of motion (ROM), and there must be a gradual emphasis on the negative phase of the work (the lowering phase of the resistance).

Types of Contractions

ISOMETRIC CONTRACTION-

Isometric contraction occurs when the distance between each end of the muscle- the origin and the insertion – remains the same even though the muscle is contraction. An observer can not see an outer movement but the person engaging in isometric contraction can feel the fiber condensing or extending. For example when you push or pull against a pole attached to the ground.

ISOTONIC CONTRACTION-

During an isotonic contraction one will observe an outer movement. Here the contraction fibers generate tension, which is greater than the load on the fibers. Isotonic contraction includes two types, eccentric contraction and concentric contraction.

ECCENTRIC CONTRACTION—

When the muscle fibers become more extended and the distance between the origin and the insertion is greater. For example, when we use the band while straightening the arm from a bent position, we will get a smooth, integrated movement that works eccentrically on the muscle.

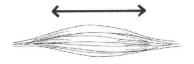

CONCENTRIC CONTRACTION

When the distance between the origin and the insertion becomes smaller. It is used in opposition to the eccentric contraction; for example, if the muscles on one side of a joint are concentrically contracting, the muscles on the other side of the joint will be eccentrically contracting.

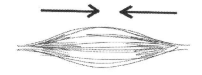

ISOMETRIC CONTRACTION

When the distance between the origin and the insertion remains the same. We will not see an outer movement, but we will sense the muscle fibers condensing or extending, giving a different quality of sensation.

MORE ABOUT ECENTRIC CONTACTION-

Eccentric contraction is a lengthening contraction. It occurs when the contracting muscle fibers become more extended and the distance between the origin and the insertion is increased. In eccentric contraction few muscle fibers are capable of contracting individually.

This puts much tension on the connective tissue, which may later relate to muscle soreness. (Asmussen1956, Fride'n et al1981, Tullson & Armstrong1981, Newham et al 1983, Fride'n 1984, Alter1988)

In found in my clinical and classroom experience, that the soreness occurred only in the early stages of the program and as the person gets stronger and more flexible using the band, the soreness is no longer a factor. Other studies completed on the subject include Cardinal & Hilsendager's (1997), who looked at ankle strength while using eccentric contraction. Rodenburg et al (1993) looked at the relations between muscle soreness and biochemical and functional outcomes of eccentric exercise. They concluded that more measures were needed at more points in time. Balnave & Thompson (1993) discussed the effects of training on eccentric exercise-induced muscle damage. Their conclusion was 'recovery of muscle function seemed to follow the same time course of adaptation as the serum muscle protein response. Training reduced muscle function impairment, suggesting that the immediate decrements in muscle function are due to a change within the muscle itself, rather than metabolic or electric alterations.' Lacerete et al (1992) explored concentric versus combined concentric-eccentric isokinetic training program. They looked at the effect on peak torque of human quadriceps rectus femoris muscle, such as when the muscle is required to contract in a set of four maximal consecutive voluntary contractions. Their findings suggest that the addition of an eccentric training component to a concentric isokinetic training program may allow greater torque gains regardless of the velocity.

Types of Stretching

PASSIVE—an outside force is pushing or pulling while you remain relaxed.

PASSIVE/ACTIVE—same as number 1, except at the peak of the stretch you will be holding the position for a few seconds.

ACTIVE/ASSISTED—you will stretch to your limits and then an outside force will continue to stretch further. Care, knowledge, and sensitivity must be exercised to avoid tearing a muscle or tendon.

ACTIVE—you use your own muscle power without outside aid. Active stretching can either be

STATIC, with a slow steady stretch (as in yoga), or it can be

BALLISTIC, with the muscle bouncing or "popping" over the joint.

The approach taken in this book is the active-static stretch. Some research may show that a combination of static and ballistic stretching could be the most beneficial, but ballistic stretching is known to cause injuries, especially to the tendons. It is very hard on the joints. My goal is to "create space" in the joints, which will avoid grinding and tension. Therefore, static stretching with the aid of the Thera-Band® will safely give you the results you are looking for—and much more.

Another method of stretching is P.N.F, Propioreceptor Neuromuscular Facilitation, which is a type of stretching developed in the nineteen forties and designed to treat people with paralysis. The method uses the body's primitive muscle reflexes. Two of the techniques are:

CONTRACT-RELAX: You contract the muscle you want to stretch for 15 seconds. The Golgi tendon registers the tension increase and causes autogenic inhibition, and that muscle will stretch further on the next try.

CONTRACT-RELAX-AGONIST-CONTRACT (CRAC): You move the muscle into a starting position. Once there, you should be holding the contraction for 20 seconds. You pause for a second and then you contract the opposing muscle to be stretched, by moving the muscle to a stronger stretch.

Planes of Movement

One of the ways to analyze muscle function and movement is to isolate the three distinct planes of the body:

FRONTAL PLANE—division from one side of the body to the other, creating separate front and back regions; movement in this plane is sagittal (directly forward and backward).

SAGITTAL PLANE—division through the center of the body, creating two symmetrical halves; movement in this plane is frontal (with the face forward; i.e., lateral bend to the side).

HORIZONTAL PLANE—division of the body at the waistline into upper and lower regions; Movement in this plane is rotation.

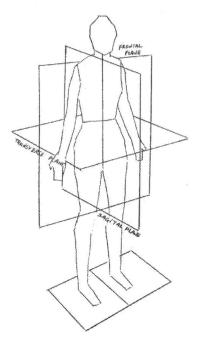

Some Principles for Muscle Movement

The body includes w network of around 600-700 muscles. They brake down to three major types, the cardiac (relating to the heart) visceral (in the wall of internal structures), and skeletal (attached to bones). Our muscles are either voluntary or involuntary. Voluntary muscles are the ones designed to controlled movement by using our nervous system.

All arranged in a sac like wrapped, the fascia, in different sizes and shapes ready for the neurologic input asking for movement. Skeletal muscles contract according to the graded strength principle. It means that they contract with varying degrees of strength at different times. That enables us to adjust from lifting a pen to lifting a full suitcase. This is different from the all or none rule on the fiber contraction level. Skeletal muscles almost always work in groups. There is a coordinated action of several muscles for performing a movement. That means that when a prime muscle is contracting an antagonist muscle will relax. At time there are muscles that work in a synergy to help the prime mover.

This allows a dynamic tension, meaning - if the front of the body has to flax forward to pick a bag, the muscles in the back of the body have to let go, and even extend to allow that motion.

Gravity -pay attention to the verticality of the body meaning- the skeleton needs to be aligned. In some of the exercises I work against gravity using it in a dynamic way (leg work) I tried to honor these principle, here and created movements that combined muscle groups, as we need them for daily function rather then trying to artificially isolate them.

By doing so, the movements keep the natural joint motion which in return help keep, or restore joint health.

Body Alignment

Body alignment is the habitual way in which we each maintain our own body placement. Personal body alignment can be acquired through:

- Imitation (i.e., baby watching parents),
- Use or misuse of the body of which you are unaware (i.e., sitting for hours in a chair),
- Genetic defects (i.e., one leg longer than the other).

Good alignment is crucial to maintaining good health. It provides the appropriate starting point for any movement or posture desired. Proper alignment will also eliminate unnecessary stress on muscles, tendons, bones, and joints; therefore, standing will be easier, breathing will be freer, and movement will be possible in any direction.

Achieving good alignment means that unnecessary stress on the body is eliminated and the body can now be maintained upright in space, against gravity. The bones are stacked one on top of another in a way that the weight will fall through the bones that are specifically designed to carry the body's weight.

The nervous system and the supporting deep muscles, fascia, tendons, and ligaments will give the support to free the muscles for movement. When the bones support the body weight, the muscles can relax, and more easily contract when movement is desired. See Ida P Rolf, Ph.D. Rolfing the Integration of Human Structures.

Another aspect of good alignment is the distribution of balance on weight-bearing and weight-transferring areas of the skeleton. You need to find the right relationship between muscles that work as the mover and the opposing antagonist muscles, thus enabling you to move with ease and efficiency. For example, the muscles on all four sides of your lower leg work together in harmony (which functions in weight-transference), so your ankle and foot can move as they were intended to (weight-bearing).

Personally I believe that one of the ways we are expressed in the world is in the posture and alignment we create through our lifetime. Our feelings, attitudes, and internal conversations about the outer world is one factor that creates our posture (heritage, repetitive movements, injuries, body structure and such, are the others). My goal is to give you the opportunity to view posture as dynamic, as transition from posture to posture that allows us to be alive in our body alignment. Alive—meaning the awareness of who we choose to be mentally and spiritually that express itself in the physical body.

Looking at Your Own Body Alignment:

When you check your body for good alignment you will divide the body into right and left sides, comparing size and length of different body parts. You will also divide the body into front/back, and lower/upper relationships. The main body parts to check are:

- The feet,
- Achilles tendon alignment to the center of the calf muscle.
- Front of center kneecap aligned with the space between second and third toe.
- Behind the knee, looking at the muscle bulk.
- Front and back of pelvis
- Skin creases along side of the torso
- Ribs
- Spine deviation from center: forward/backwards and side deviation that can be in a c shape all to the right, all to the left or in an s shape crossing from right to left, left to right.
- Shoulders level as well as ears level.

Compare one side with the other, looking for such conditions as one shoulder higher than the other, one knee turned inward, or one inner thigh muscle more or less developed than the other. As you practice observing, you will "develop an eye" for recognizing areas of muscles that are defined, as opposed to areas of weakness and low tonicity; areas with "moving energy" and areas with no "life."

The relationship between posture and skeletal structure is alive and ongoing throughout your lifetime. Most people find that their bodily structure mirrors and profoundly influences their posture. By opening up an awareness of body language—that is, by paying attention to how you do things: how you stand, sit, step, or adjust your balance—you will avoid body stiffening, inflexibility, imbalance, and/or pain in the soft tissues become more dynamic. As a result, you will avoid bodily stiffening, inflexibility, imbalance, and/or pain in the soft tissues. You will become more dynamic.

Examples of Common of Misalignments

1. Neck that protrudes forward causing stress on the cervical vertebras. This causes the back (posterior) neck muscles to be contracted continuously; the anterior neck muscles will be long and weak, causing imbalance that may lead to injury and pain.

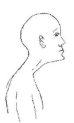

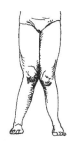

2. Knees that are turned in more than the feet. The stress will then be placed on the tendons and ligaments on the lateral aspects of the knee and the inner/outer thigh muscles will be under stress. The side muscles in the lower leg may build enough stress for you to sense pain.

3. Feet with fallen arches. This puts undue stress on the lateral aspect of the ankle and increases the chance for injury.

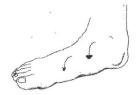

The human body is not a static structure; it is very dynamic and constantly moving (our center of gravity is high, 1-2 inches below the navel). In order to adapt to each new position, good alignment continuously changes, as the body keeps moving. Therefore, when thinking about posture, we should not relate it just to any one fixed position, but to the relationships among body parts as they are moving. When you are able to move harmoniously from one point to another with the required effort, you are on the path towards better alignment. For example, picture yourself sitting with your legs crossed in front of you. If you are unable to maintain the position for a long time, you may suffer from any of the following deviations:

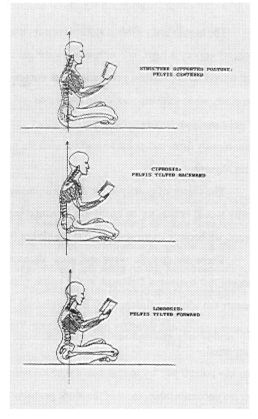

1. Your weight may not be on both sitting bones, and or either in front of or behind them;

2. You may not be breathing down into your lower abdominal or lower back (floating ribs), but may be breathing shallowly in your upper chest only;

3. Your weight may not be falling through the front of the second lumber vertebra; or

4. Your chest may be sinking back while your neck is pushed forward.

By attending to habits like these, finding the place were the bones carry the body weight and the muscles are free for movement you will improve your body alignment.

Many tests can measure and determine if you are in proper alignment. The Thomas test measures tightness of the pelvis (illiopsoas and rectus femoris). The Ober test measures adductor tightness (ITB and gluteal). The Tripod test measures the tightness of the hamstring muscle group and it effect on the position (tilt) of the pelvis.

The key point is this: If you try to maintain a position that seems to be good posture to you, but yet you are uncomfortable, your muscles are probably doing most of the work. You might not have enough skeletal support. Improvement will come when you start viewing your alignment as dynamic

Breathing

Any time that we find ourselves under a physical demand, we may become somewhat aware of the way we are breathing. Our breathing patterns tend to change to adapt with our emotions; for example, we breathe differently when we feel fear, hesitation, surprise, joy, happiness, or even when something simply interests us. People of different professions like singing and dancing often have specific breathing techniques they must learn. We breathe differently as our body is in different positions—lying on one side (which puts pressure on one lung), sitting, standing, or even hanging upside-down.

Think of the rib cage as a container for the thoracic cavity, which holds the lungs. The heart sits in between them, more to the left side of center; this would explain why the left lung is slightly smaller than the right one, and why the bronchus of the left lung has only two main branches instead of three, like the right one has.

The lungs are an organ that helps our body absorb the oxygen into our cells when we inhale, and gets rid of excess carbon dioxide when we exhale.

The breathing movement occurs in the muscles surrounding the lungs. The main muscle, which initiates the breathing action and also performs 80% of the work, is the diaphragm—a strong, thin muscle located between the thoracic and abdominal cavities. It is attached to the lower border of the rib cage (anterior) and all the way around to the spine (posterior). On an inhalation, the diaphragm contracts by flattening downwards into the abdomen, enlarging the thoracic cavity, which creates an atmospheric pressure and allows air to flow from the outside of the body to the inside.

Another muscle that contracts during the inhalation is the intercostal muscle located between the ribs. When one takes a very deep inhalation, or forcefully exhales, other muscles may also be involved such as those around the shoulder, neck, and back.

The exhalation is a reverse process of what happens during the inhalation; the muscles stop the contraction and relax, and the air simply flows out of the trachea and the mouth as the abdominal and thoracic muscles and organs return to their original positions.

Breathing is a key to well-being in many belief systems; not just physically, but also mentally and emotionally. Each one of us can improve the way we breathe in order to benefit our health.

One of the things I stress most in this book is for you to keep your breathing pattern steady and constant as you exercise, using the whole thoracic cavity, in front, in back, and along the sides, from the sternum down into the pelvis. Notice when your rhythm changes; it may be an indication of difficulty or an anticipation of effort. Check your body alignment and muscle relaxation between repetitions to be certain that there is no tension or exertion. If you find that you are starting to hold your breath, STOP!

Go back to the beginning of the exercise, and then start to exhale as you perform the movement.

Adjust your workout to your abilities and needs, so that when you are finished, you will feel invigorated rather than exhausted.

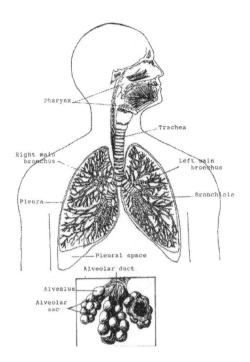

Head and Tail/bone Relationship

The head and the tail/bone are at the two ends of the spine; therefore, it is very important that they work together. From the time that you were a baby, they each responded to the other naturally when you moved; for example, as you arched your neck and head, trying to crawl on your stomach in prone position,(and later on your hands and knees). Chiropractors tend to utilize that principle in their work. This relationship can be seen when you work from the all fours position. As you arch the spine, both the head and the tail/bone will be directed up toward the ceiling. As the spine curves upward, both the head and tail/bone will be directed down toward the floor. This is also true for a cat stretching as it is waking up.

For more information on the relationship of the head and tail/bone, particularly during infancy and childhood, refer to Bonnie Bainbridge Cohen's studies at the School for Body-Mind Centering, as recorded in the Bibliography and Suggested Reading section at the end of the book

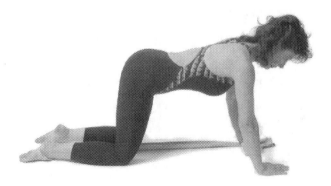

Awareness

Feldenkrais in his book Awareness Through Movement, page 50. Says "Awareness is consciousness together with a realization of what is happening within it or what is going on within ourselves while we are conscious." Having an adequate awareness would mean that we know what it is we are doing while we are in the act.

Awareness is the strongest tool I know of which we have for relearning and reeducating ourselves. Awareness is the extra ingredient we should add to moving, thinking, sensing, and feeling. We learn to move as infants by imitation. We do movements mostly the way we learned them, and get into habits. Here we are together to improve some parts of the habitual ways we move in. This will enable us to access the knowing of how we do our movements, with out strain and force.

Gaining awareness will give us the ability to choose. It will also give us an access to the body mind connection we all feel and know we have. For example, changing our body posture when we feel fear will result in altering our feeling to some extent. Change of mental focus can effect the intensity of pain; and positive thoughts can alter our mental state.

The avenues to body mind connection are many. I hope that the journey through the physical realm, I bring here, will give you an access to finding your connection. Even though the intent here is to achieve a stronger and more flexible body, if you do the exercises with intention, attention and awareness (mindfulness) you will get closer to your full potential finding improvement in both body & mind.

1   Interconnections

One hot summer afternoon to escape from domestic drudgery, I went to a movie little realizing the intellectual work out in store for me. The movie "Mind Walk" was a debate between three very different but very cerebral types. Besides forcing me to think about major dilemmas of our time, it introduced me to a new term important in physics: interconnections. As a result of this term and the way it was used in the movie, I now find myself looking at people, things and places with somewhat new awareness. I can now perceive how all of these relate to one another through vibrations of energy. I am discovering truth and comfort in knowing that I am related to all that I see, hear, feel and touch (and in more subtle ways the silver-mercury sitting and relating to my teeth, the material I am wearing, etc.). The film "Mind Walk" featured three distinct types with a different outlook on life. There was the physicist, her outlook being scientific yet holistic and avant guard, the pragmatic politician and finally the poet/political speechwriter representing the arts. A bridge is affected between the scientist and politician. It remained for the poet to remind us of the absolute necessity of emotions for a full, complete understanding of life function. So there it is: function, force and feeling, all integrated, all interconnected. Interconnections.

2

It is possible to actually believe that dancers or athletes are somehow more than moral when we see them in competition or performance. Their abilities may amaze us. However, behind the outward appearances, pain and injury are often the price of excellence.

We sometimes forget the human structure—the shape of the joints, the length of the ligaments and tendons—and try to reach the aesthetic beauty that the culture and tradition of classical ballet has set for us, as well as the speed and agility of many sports. By knowing the body movement capability from within, along with the realistic capabilities we may be able to minimize the agony. We should "create space" in the joints before movement and use deep muscles in a three dimension fashion.

3

Once, while serving in the Israeli army, I was in an army settlement that was soon to be turned into a civil community. I took a late walk one night outside the security fence, not thinking of the danger or the consequences.

The next morning, there was a gathering of people in the central dining hall, and their emotions were very stirred. I soon learned that the Bedouin who walked the borders that morning had found footprints. Just by looking at them, he could tell that a five foot, two inch tall female who was bout 20 years old left them. He Knew There was nothing left for me to do. So with a smile and a guilty conscience I stepped forward.

I then spent years looking to discover even part of what he never forgot from his years of living in the desert and being one with nature and its courses.

4

Do I need my hands to get up from a chair?

It depends from which end you are looking at it. For a young child, it is a matter of fact. For an elderly person, it may be a major effort. (Just look at all the T.V. advertisements for automatic chairs that lift you up from them!)

As I see the task, it all boils down to a shift of weights and correct timing; it is not a matter of being "strong" enough to pull yourself up, but of how to use your body correctly. So–

Sit at the edge of a chair with your sitting bones touching the edge and your feet flat on the floor about as far apart as your pelvic width. Start playing with you upper body weight, shifting it forward and backward, then side to side. Find your personnel comfort zone. Find when the discomfort starts to "creep in." Notice that when you shift your weight forward, your heels dig in to the floor to a full contact. What happens then to your abdominal muscles?

Now pay attention to what happens to your neck and chin as you shift your weight forward. Can you feel the curvature in your neck also going forward?

When you shift enough weight forward, your pelvis will elevate and rotate a bit forward, the curvature in your neck will increase, the weight will be over your feet (through the second toe), and you will be lifting out of the chair to a "chimpanzee position." From there to an upright standing position, the distance is short.

5

I remember days in college that it was just "too much" and I "needed air," and I would go to one of my favorite places to escape from stress; the beach. But even while I was there, my interest in human movement was still present.

For example, I would find a rock to sit on and I would watch people as they walked by. At other times, I used to walk along the beach myself. I would follow behind a certain person, observing their body alignment as they walked, and then I would look at the footprints they made in the sand to see how their weight was distributed as they moved. I soon learned to find the correlation between the two. You can learn a lot about a person simply by watching how they carry themselves.

Try "people watching" sometime. It can be amusing, and you may find that it is rather amazing as well. Perhaps it might even make you stop and think about your own alignment and the way you move. If someone were watching you, what would they see? What kind of stories does your own walk tell about you?

6

Have you ever watched a mother and daughter walking together in the mall, a father and son walking into a restaurant to find a seat, or any other combination of family members, for that matter? When you watch children, you will usually find a mirror, a duplication of the parents' own choices of movement patterns. For generations, parents have unknowingly passed their own movement compensations onto their children. A child's internal temp; rhythm; swing of the hip; posture; use or misuse of the swing of the arms and the shoulders; back rotation; the shift the weight on their legs—all seem to have been unconsciously learned from the parent since infancy.

It would appear that human beings have forsaken many of their natural instincts for movement somewhere along the way. And still, with all the intelligence mankind has gained, we still have to learn by watching our models, and by our own trial and error, to sit , walk, speak, etc.

#7

I have a friend who once worked as a massage therapist. Then, while on vacation, she had a tobogganing accident and broke her 10th vertebra, right at her mid-back. The doctors who performed her surgery fused together the vertebras around the injured one.

Afterward, she asked hem to prescribe physical therapy and machine work for her to strengthen her back, but their answer to her was not to waste her time; she would not walk again.

The community came to her side to help her. People from all sorts of body work professions volunteered their time and effort to work with her, believing it was possible to re channel her movement paths along different routes of the body, in order to bypass the nerve damage.

#8 Have you ever watched a baby? Brand new human beings are always in motion. Watch the big movements of the baby, forever kicking his legs, rolling over and over, or scooting across the floor. Watch the small movements of a baby calming herself to sleep, or the even smaller movements of a sleeping baby, as he breathes with the whole diaphragm, lifting and expanding the rib cage up to the outer rotation of the arms before he exhales. Why then do we freeze, stiffen, and reduce our own possibilities for movement as we go through life?

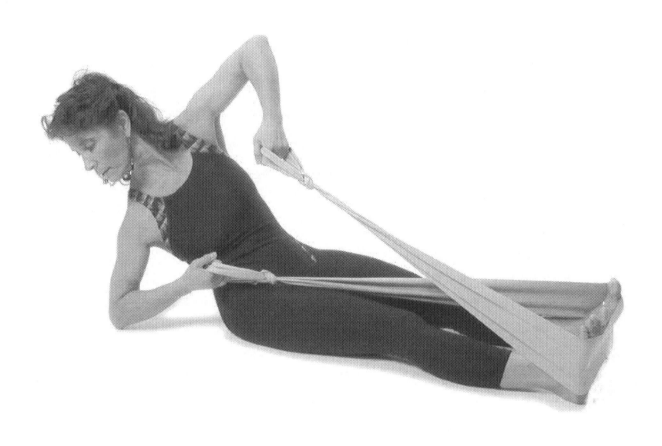

Chapter 2

EXERCISES

PART 1

CENTER OF THE BODY

"AWARENESS IS THE HIGHEST STAGE IN MAN'S DEVELOPMENT,
AND WHEN IT IS COMPLETE IT MAINTAINS A HARMONIOUS
'RULE' OVER THE BODY'S ACTIVITIES."

Moshe Feldenkrais
The Elusive Obvious (1981:70)

MAIN GROUPS OF MUSCLES INVOLVED IN PART 1

MUSCLES OF THE ABDOMINAL:

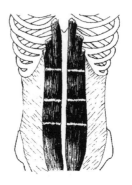

1. Rectus abdominalis

2. Obliquus externus abdominalis

3. Obliquus internus abdominalis

4. Transversus abdominalis

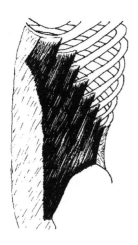 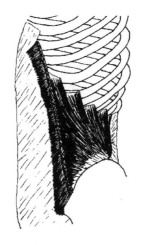

MUSCLES OF THE BACK:

1. Quadratus lumborum

QUADRATUS LUMBORUM

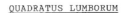

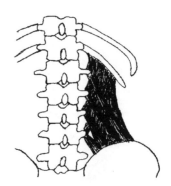

2. Erector spina

3. Splenius muscles

(Cervicis capitis)

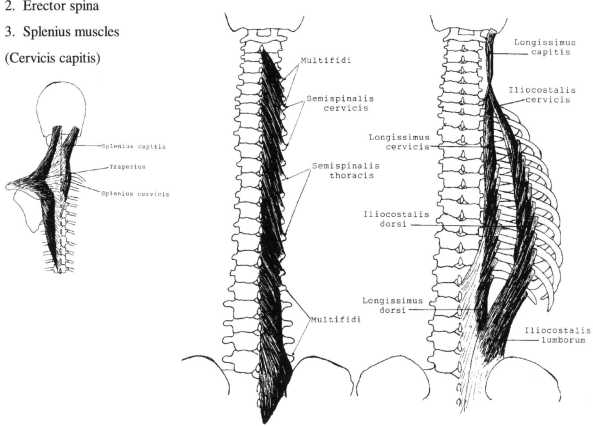

Splenius capitis

Trapezius

Splenius cervicis

Multifidi

Semispinalis cervicis

Semispinalis thoracis

Multifidi

Longissimus capitis

Iliocostalis cervicis

Longissimus cervicis

Iliocostalis dorsi

Longissimus dorsi

Iliocostalis lumborum

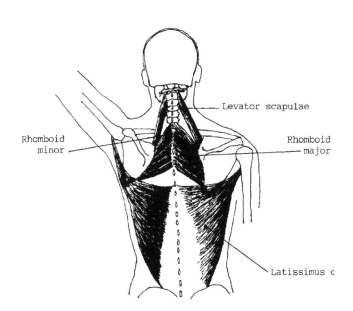

Levator scapulae

Rhomboid minor

Rhomboid major

Latissimus d

4. Transversospinalis Semispinalis (layer1)

B. Multifidi (layer 2)

C. Rotators (layer 3)

5. Interspinalis

6. Intertransversarii

HIP FLEXOR: Iliopsoas

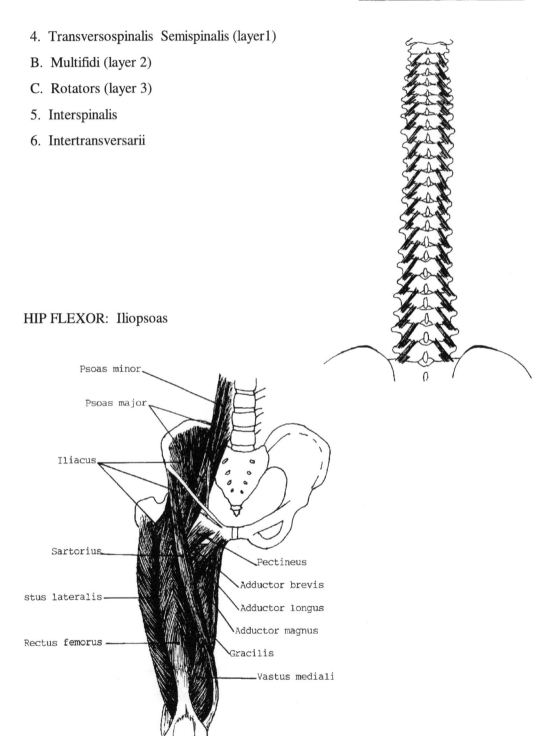

Psoas minor

Psoas major

Iliacus

Sartorius

stus lateralis

Rectus femorus

Pectineus

Adductor brevis

Adductor longus

Adductor magnus

Gracilis

Vastus mediali

I. ABDOMINALS: THE ICE CREAM SCOOPER

POSITION: Sit on the floor with your legs in front of you and point your toes toward the ceiling.

BAND: Place the center of band on the soles of the feet, across the metatarsal. Cross each side of the band in front of the shins and hold in the opposite hand at a point on the band that will provide you with the appropriate amount of resistance. NOTE: A. If your feet tend to turn in or out, wrap the band once around the feet to hold them steady and aligned before crossing the band in front of the shins.

B. The knees are softened slightly to prevent hyper extension. If needed, you may place a towel, small pillow, or other support underneath them.

C. The elbows are pointed out, arms are lifted, and shoulders are pressed down. Think of the back widening, so that the latissimus dorsi muscle is being used throughout the exercise

EXERCISE: 1. Lower your torso back toward the floor against the resistance of the band. The curve of the spine will initiate from the spine's base, and in turn, will affect each successive vertebra. Your head will be last to bend, but it will not begin to curve until it is inevitable.

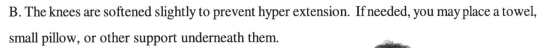

2. As you tilt your pelvis, imagine you are scooping out the contents of your abdominal.

3. Continue the scooping motion all the way down until your shoulders reach the ground.

4. Without resting your weight back on the floor, slowly return to the starting position by reversing the curving order of the vertebra, starting with your head. Use the same scooping sensation, and breath evenly.

5. Once your head is directly in line over your tail/bone, start to straighten your back with the movement initiating from the tail/bone and continuing like a wave through each vertebra of the spine up to the head.

6. Roll down as in number 1. On the way up once your head is in line above your pelvis, initiate the

straightening of the spine from the center of your back instead of at the base. Both the head and tail/bone will arrive at their final positions at the same time.

7. Repeat. Straightening of the spine will be initiated from the head.

VARIATION: Repeat number 7 while holding both ends of the band in one hand as you roll the spine down, and return. Hold the other hand out beside you. Be sure to keep both sides of the body equal as you do the exercises.

II. ABDOMINALS: ROTATION

POSITION: Sit with your legs in front of you.

BAND: Place the center of band on the soles of the feet, across the metatarsal. Cross each side of the band in front of the shins and hold in the opposite hand at a point on the band that will provide you with the appropriate amount of resistance.

EXERCISE:

1. Pull your L elbow away from the R elbow as the back rotates to the L side. Your spine should be straight and as high as possible without the shoulders lifting or shrugging. Be sure you are sitting directly on top of your ischial tuberosities (the sitting bones), and the spine rotates on top of the fixed pelvis. This will isolate the rotation muscle around your spine in order to rotate to each side. Do it once fixating the legs and once allowing the leg to lengthen and shorten with the back rotation to get a whole body movement

2. Repeat number 1. Your legs should be a little wider than hip width apart. As you rotate to the L side this time, the pelvis will also be allowed to rotate; the L leg will shorten into the hip socket while the R leg seems to lengthen and grow longer (with out bending at the knee).

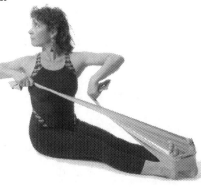

-42-

III. ABDOMINALS: COMBINATION

POSITION: Sit on the floor with your legs in front of you.

BAND: Wrap the band in the same way as in exercise I&2.

EXERCISE: (combination of 1+2)

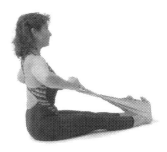

1. Curve the spine to lower your torso to the floor, initiating the movement from the base of the spine and scooping the abdominal as in the exercise I, except you will rotate the hip and back to the L side at the same time as in number 2.

2. Keep your arms and elbows at the same distance and relationship from the body as you move.

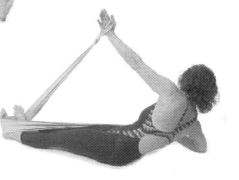

3. End up with your L elbow on the floor and your R elbow pointing 180 ° diagonally from it in the air.

4. Return to the starting position by reversing the movement, initiating by scooping and rotating.

ADVANCED:

(a) Repeat number 1, extending the L arm, forearm, and hand to a straightened position 180° from the opposite elbow at the same time that you roll the spine down to the floor, "scooping out" your abdominal.

 (b) Wrap both ends of the band around the L foot and hold the center of the band with your R hand, so your body will act in opposition. Contract your abdominal inward toward your spine as you rotate to the R side. Point the R elbow diagonally behind you as the spine lengthens down to the floor. Hold the L arm out to the side of the body.

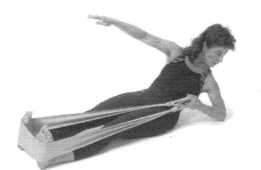

IV. ILIO-PSOAS STRETCH

POSITION: Lie on your back with the legs about hip width apart. Bend both knees and point them up toward the ceiling. Place the soles of the feet flat on the floor.

BAND: Place one end of the band around the sole of each foot; then lay it along the floor beside the body, underneath the elbows, and across the upper arms. Hold the center of the band with both hands in front of the chest.

EXERCISE:

1. Flex the feet and slowly straighten the legs by sliding the heels along the floor. Think of lengthening the legs out from the heels.

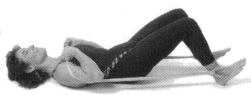

2. Hold the lower back close to the floor and do not release it throughout the   whole exercise, (Do not push it into the floor either). Use the flatten abdominal muscles to support the back.

VARIATION: After fully extending the legs, raise the head and legs few inches from the floor.

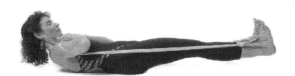

V. LEG STRETCH

POSITION: Sit with your legs in front of you.

BAND: Place the center of the band on the sole of the R
foot. Bend the knee. Place the band on each side of the R
leg and hold in each hand, or as you see in the photo.

EXERCISE:

1.   Extend your R leg and straighten your leg by
lengthening out from the heel;

   do not allow the knee joint to hyper extend backward.

2. Slowly bend your knee again.

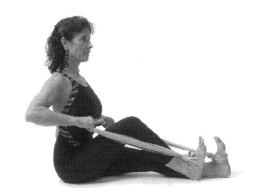

3.   Repeat, lengthening your leg a little higher each time, (4-5 repetitions). Keep your back erect.

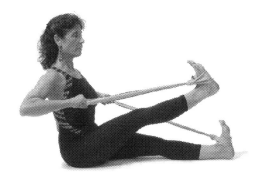
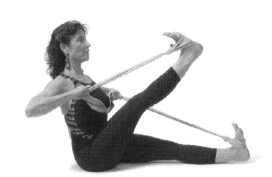

VI. SPINAL CHAIN

POSITION: Stand with your legs parallel to one another. Place your arms overhead a little wider than shoulder width apart.

BAND: Hold the band in both hands.

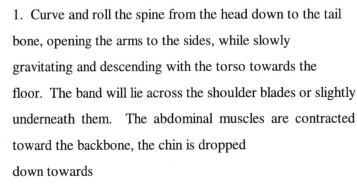

EXERCISE:

1. Curve and roll the spine from the head down to the tail bone, opening the arms to the sides, while slowly gravitating and descending with the torso towards the floor. The band will lie across the shoulder blades or slightly underneath them. The abdominal muscles are contracted toward the backbone, the chin is dropped down towards the chest, and the knees are softly bent.

2. Reaching the lowest point of your back extension, keep your arms lengthen loosely down toward the floor as your torso contracts and pulls back up towards the ceiling. Roll up in a slow count.

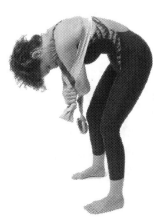

VARIATION: Same as above. Once you contract the abdominal muscles, stay in the contraction and cross your arms in front of your chest as if you were hugging yourself. Repeat it once with the R arm in front on the "hug," and once with the L arm in front. Return slowly by lifting the arms and back up at the same time.

1

When I was a dance student in college, my body was cold and stiff. One of my favorite exercises to do at the end of my warm up was to get into the yoga plow position. First, lay on your back on the floor. Bring your legs up and over your head, letting your pelvis come up as well, until your toes touch the floor above your head. The stretching sensation will expand and crawl all the way up and down the spine. When I do this, I feel like I can trace the nervous system from my spinal column through the rest of my body, just like the diagrams you see in physiology books.

2

There are no hard rules. Everyone has his or her own individual body language and develops his or her own inner logic. Maybe this is the reason there are so many techniques for "body work" and approaches to reach mind-body and soul. If none really appear to help you, then it is the time to look inside yourself and create your own. Listen to your body's messages and try to recognize how to interpret time to your best ability. The key to your own body language is always somewhere inside yourself.

#3

I have girlfriend who I have worked with for the past ten years. She is now over seventy years old. When she was fourteen, she had severe pains that prevented her from walking. The doctor found it to be degeneration of the joint between the pelvis and the leg. He fused the joint into an angle, causing the lower back to act as a joint instead.   Years later, while she was in her forties, her back gave out. The doctors had to reset the fused joint into a different angle. This wonderful woman never lost her smile. She has always continued her community work and her concern for others. Most of all, in spite of the pain and discomfort of her movement limitation, she learned new ways to cope, so she could move and dance with grace.

#4

Did you ever stop to think that if you warm up your body for physical activity by starting at the head and progressing down to your feet, a different energy results than if you had started at your feet and worked your way up to your head.

PART 2:

LOWER BODY

"TO BE ALIVE, TO KNOW LIFE, IS TO BREATHE. TO BREATHE IS TO MOVE, TO MOVE IS TO CHANGE. MOVEMENT IS FUNDAMENTAL TO LIFE."

FROM MARIECHILD, DIANE (1987)
THE INNER DANCE, FREEDOM, CA.;
THE CROSSING PRESS

THE MAIN MUSCLE GROUPS USED IN PART 2.

MUSCLES FOR HIP ADDUCTION

1. Pectineus
2. Gracilis
3. Adductor longus
4. Adductor brevis
5. Adductor magnus

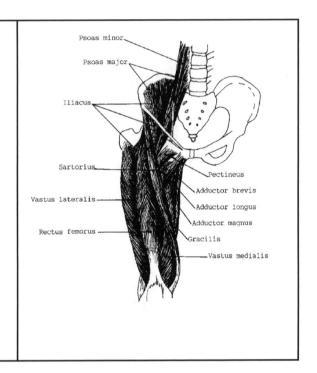

MUSCLES FOR HIP ABDUCTION

1. Tensor fascia lata
2. Gluteus medius
3. Gluteus minimus
4. The six deep rotators
   A. Piriformis
   B. Superior gemellus
   C. Obterator internus
   D. Inferior gemellus
   E. Obturator externus
   F. Quadratus femoris

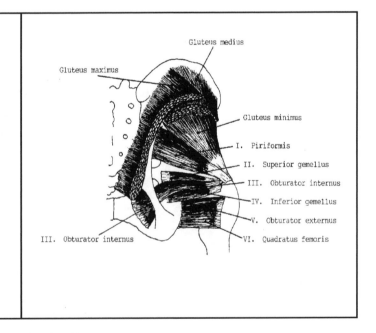

MUSCLE GROUP OF THE POSTERIOR
THIGH:
  Hamstring
1. Biceps femoris
2. Semitendinosus
3. Semimembranosus

MUSCLE GROUP OF THE ANTERIOR
THIGH:
  Quadriceps
1. Rectus femoris
2. Vastus lateralis
3. Vastus medialis
4. Vastus intermedium
SEE PAGE 53

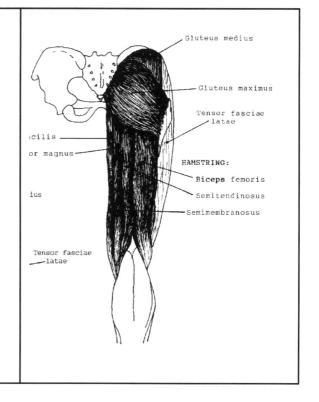

MUSCLES FOR INWARD ROTATION OF
THE HIP
1. Tensor fascia lata
2. Gluteus minimus (in femur abduction)
3. Semitendinosus
4. Gracilis

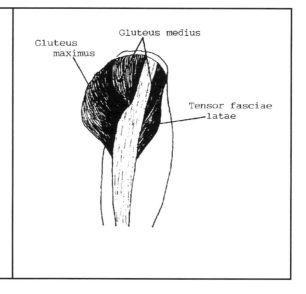

MUSCLES FOR OUTWARD
ROTATION OF THE HIP
1. Gluteus medius (in hip abduction)
2. Gluteus maximus
3. The six deep lateral rotator muscles
A. Piriformis
B. Gemellus superior
C. Gemellus inferior
D. Obturator externous
E. Obturator internous
F. Quadratus femoris
4. Iliopsoas (in thigh flexion)
5. Sartorius (in thigh flexion)
6. Biceps femoris
7. Adductor brevis (in hip adduction)
8. Adductor magnus (in hip adduction)

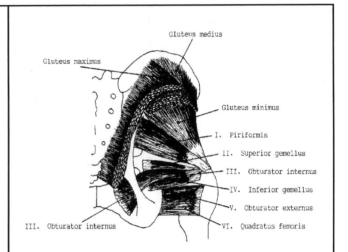

MUSCLE FOR HIP AND KNEE
FLEXION:

Sartorius

MUSCLE FOR KNEE FLEXION:

Popliteus

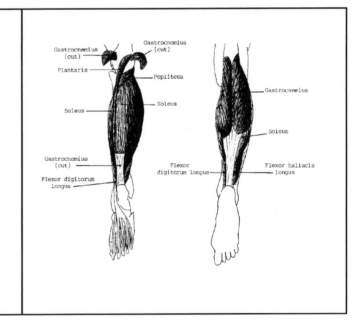

MUSCLES OF THE CALF AND FOOT	MUSCLES FOR DORSI FLEXION OF THE FOOT
1. Plantar flexors	1. Extensor digitorum longus
2. Gastrocnemius	2. Extensor hallucis longus
3. Flexor digitorum longus	3. Tibialis anterior
4. Flexor hallucis longus	
5. Peroneus longus	
6. Peroneus brevis	
7. Plantaris 8. Soleus	
9. Tibialis posterior	

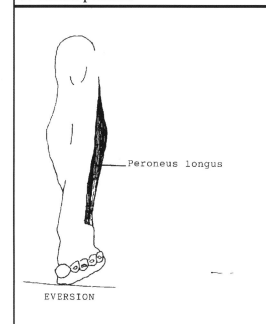

Peroneus longus

EVERSION

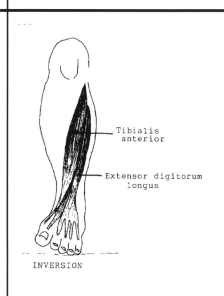

Tibialis anterior

Extensor digitorum longus

INVERSION

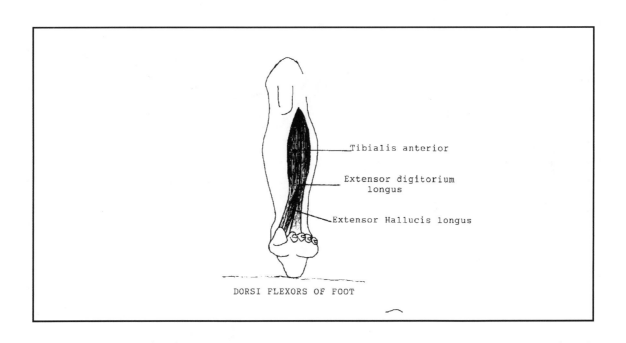

Tibialis anterior

Extensor digitorium
longus

Extensor Hallucis longus

DORSI FLEXORS OF FOOT

-54-

I. ANTIGRAVITY LEGWORK

POSITION: Lie on your back with both legs held at a 90° angle up in the air. By keeping the legs directly above the hip, you will work the leg extensor, especially those behind the knee.

BAND: Place the ends of the band around the sole of each foot, crossed in front of the shins, and held in the hands at a point on the band that will provide you with the appropriate amount of resistance. Place your elbows and upper arms are on the floor beside you.

NOTE: Sensing where 90° is in this position may be difficult; most people tend to have their legs leaning too far forward or backward.

Therefore, it would be a good idea to do exercises in this position with a mirror nearby, or better yet, with the legs up against a wall.

EXERCISES:

1. (a) Slowly, bend the knees, creating an imaginary straight line between your toes and your navel. Do not let your legs lean toward your face. Be sure your spine remains in another straight line from head to tail/bone, and your pelvis does not tilt as the knees bend.

    (b) Keeping the feet flexed, push the heels upward to slowly straighten the knees. The center of the kneecaps should be on an imaginary line to your second-third toe. You should feel a stretch from the heels to the tail/bone in opposite directions (Make sure you do not push your knees backwards).

2. THE DIAMOND:

    (a) Straighten your legs in a parallel position with the sides of your feet together.

    (b) Keeping your heels together, rotate your legs outward from the hip socket into a first position. Do not let your legs turn out more at your feet than at your hip joints.

(c) Starting in this turned out first position, repeat exercise 1. As you bend your knees, do not let your feet to turn out more than your knees or hips.

3. DIAGONAL ARROW:

(a) Bend the knees in a plie' in first position, as in exercise 2.

(b) Straighten the R leg in a diagonal to the R side. Both R and L feet remain flexed.

(c) Bend the R knee: return to first position diamond shape.

(d) Do the same with your L leg.

4. Repeat exercise 3, straightening both knees diagonally out to the sides at the same time.

5. (a) Start with your legs in a parallel second position, a little wider than hip width apart.

(b) Bend both legs to a diamond.

(c) Straighten by lengthening out from the heels. (This exercise is the same as exercise 1, except it is in second position, and in parallel.)

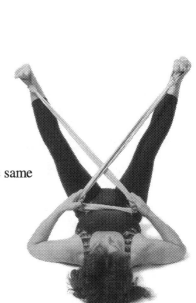

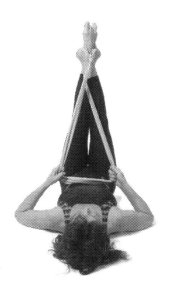

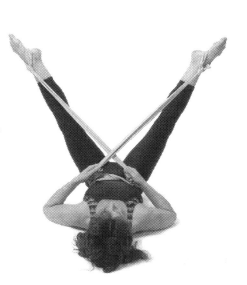

6. SCISSORS:

(a) Turn out legs are crossed one in front of the other in a fifth position in the air (or against a wall).

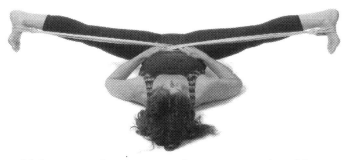

(b) Use a wide scissors kick to open the   legs to a second position.

(c) Return to fifth position again, alternating which foot is in front each time.

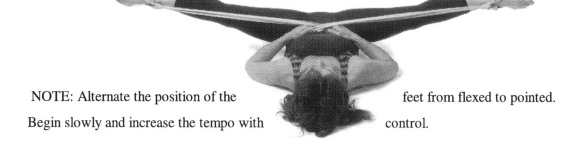

NOTE: Alternate the position of the   feet from flexed to pointed. Begin slowly and increase the tempo with   control.

II. ADVANCED ANTI GRAVITY LEGWORK

POSITION: Lie on your back, legs at 90° in the air (or against a wall).

BAND: The band should be in the same position as in exercise I.

EXERCISE:

1. Instead of exercise 6 in ANTI-GRAVITY LEGWORK, open the legs into a wide second position, toes facing the floor, without tilting the pelvis off of the floor

2. Bend your knees, turning your legs out even more.

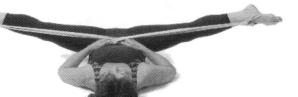

3.   Straighten your legs by lengthening out from the heels.

4. Repeat,   bending your knees in the wide position four times.

5. Lift both legs slowly as you return to the starting position.

6. Lower one leg to the floor directly to the side, keeping   the other leg up in the air; then return. Flex/point the feet as desired.

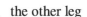

7. Repeat, lowering one leg directly in front of you; then return.

NOTE: You will be unable to complete this exercise if your legs are against a wall.

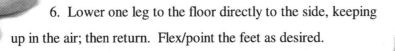

III. THE STORK LEGWORK

POSITION: Stand with your feet about hip width apart. Bend your knees slightly.

BAND: Place both ends of the band are on the R foot. Spread the center of the band over your L shoulder.

EXERCISES: Begin each exercise by lifting the flexed R foot to knee height.

1. TENDU:

Extend your R leg 45° diagonal forward, in a parallel. Your heel should touch the floor. Allow your hip to rise and sink as you do the movement.

2. Repeat number 1, fixating the pelvis; the leg will work separately from the hip.

3. DEVELOPPE':

(a) Develop your R leg to a full extension in the air with a flexed foot. Do not allow your hip to rise or the torso to sink into the pelvis in order to achieve more height. The height of your leg will depend upon your flexibility.

(b) Lower the flexed foot to the floor in a parallel position, 45° diagonal.

4. Extend the flexed R foot 45° diagonal, leg is parallel and to the side, foot flexed. (Most people will not be able to open their leg exactly to the side of the body, so you may open your leg on a diagonal if necessary.)

5. (a) Extend the flexed R foot behind you with your heel leading.

(b) Return to parallel first position with your toes leading.

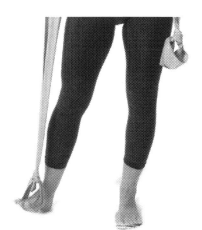

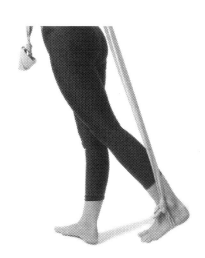

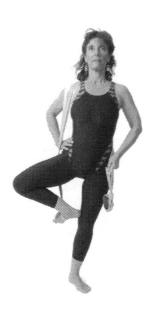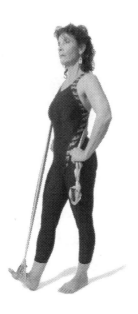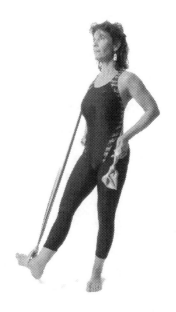

6. Repeat exercises 1-5 with the R thigh turned out instead of parallel.

7. Repeat all the above exercises (with R leg in turned in and turned out positions) with the R foot pointed instead of flexed.

NOTE:

(a) Throughout the exercises, the supporting leg is extremely important, and you need to "climb" out of it.

(b) Make sure your knee is not hyper-extended.

(c) The tail/bone should be directed down to the floor, do not "tuck".

(d) The sitting bones must stay at the same height from the floor and must be on the same level as well.

IV. LYING ON ONE SIDE

POSITION: Lie on one side of your body. Bend the lower leg, and flex the toes, so they can be braced against the floor for support. Extend the upper leg. Make sure the hip muscles and the abdominal muscles initiate the movement. Support your body, so it will not roll forward or backward. Try to keep the lower ribs closed and slightly off the floor. Be especially careful your ribs do not release when you execute a movement to the back while in this position. Instead, both sides of the ribs should be aligned with one side directly on top of the other.

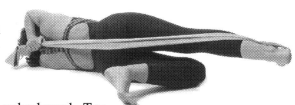

BAND: Attach both ends of the band to the upper foot. Then, stretch the band along the side of the body and behind the back. Hold the center of the band behind your neck with both hands.

NOTE: If this position is uncomfortable for you, you may hold the band by spreading it over your upper shoulder and stabilizing it with the upper hand.

EXERCISE:

1. Flex your upper foot , parallel to the floor, and at no more than three inches high.

2. Without using a large movement, lengthen your upper leg out of the hip socket. Then, shorten the leg back into the hip socket.

NOTE: Work with the hip, not the leg.

3. Turn your toes and the knee of the upper leg down toward the floor to work the tensor fascia lata. First, allow your hip to roll forward and back with the leg movement. Then, fixate the hip to isolate the leg.

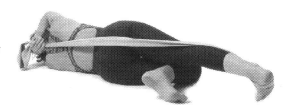

4. (a) Keeping the knee of the upper leg forward,

    lift your leg until it is slightly higher than the hip.

   (b) At that height, rotate the leg in and out.

   (c) Roll the hip at first, with the leg movement .

   (d) Then, isolate the movement of the leg from the hip.

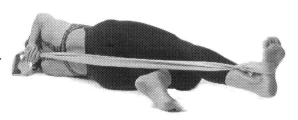

5. Turn your upper leg out, so your toes and knees will face the ceiling.

6. Lift the upper leg up as far to the side as you can, fixating the lower leg to the floor.

 NOTE: (a) Shorten the band to achieve the resistance that is right or you; then lower the upper leg back down to the bent lower leg.

(b) Do this exercise once with your upper foot flexed; then pointed.

7.   Repeat number 4. The upper leg should be in parallel position with toes and knee forward. This will limit the height the leg can rise. Once you reach the maximum height, do small pulsing motions, gently raising and lowering the leg in order to strengthen the abductors. Do this exercise once with the upper foot flexed; then pointed.

8. (a) Lift the upper leg directly in front of your body, keeping the foot at about three inches off the floor. How high you raise your leg in front of you depends on your flexibility, as long as you do not disturb your proper alignment.

(b) Shorten the band.

(c) Return the leg to the beginning position.

 NOTE: Do this exercise with the leg in parallel position--once with the foot flexed, then pointed.

9. Repeat number 8 with the leg in turned out position--once with the foot flexed, then pointed.

10. Repeat number 8 with the leg turned in, toes down toward the floor in

an everted ("sickled") position once with the foot flexed, then pointed.

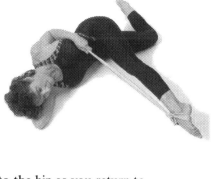

11. (a) Extend your leg in parallel to maximum extension in front of you.

    (b) Lengthen the upper leg out of the hip as the

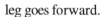

leg goes forward.

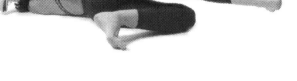

        (c) Shorten the leg into the hip as you return to the starting position.

        (d) Allow your hip to move forward and backward with the leg.

12. (a) Hold the band as before or stretch the band over your opposite shoulder on the ground

NOTE:

(a) Use the position which is more comfortable for you.

(b) Lift your upper leg toward the ceiling.

(c) Bend your knee slightly behind your body to create an arched shape.

(d) Move the thigh of your upper leg behind your body slightly, as if someone had pulled your foot.

        (e) Keep the shape of the leg, but open the angle of the knee wider.

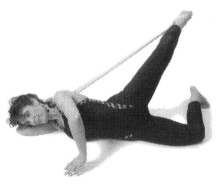

        (f) Lift and lower the entire leg as a single unit to maintain the relationship of the thigh to the lower leg.

13. (a) Bend your knee of the upper leg into an arched position as in number 12.

(b) Straighten your leg directly behind you in a long straight line by pushing outward from the heel.

(c) Bend your leg slowly as you return to the starting position.

14. (a) Begin in the same attitude position as in number 12 and 13.

(b) Swing your upper leg gently from a position with the upper thigh turned out (and the foot touching the other knee) to a position with the upper thigh turned in (and the foot in the air behind the body).

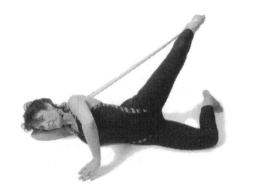 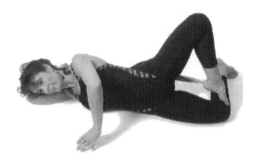

NOTE: Your knee acts as an axis so be sure the thigh and knee remain on the same level as you raise and lower your foot and lower leg. Always stay in control.

POSITION: Lie on one side with your upper leg straightened and your lower leg bent at the knee as in the exercise IV.

BAND: Attach both ends of the band to the upper foot. Stretch the band along the side of the body and behind the back. Hold the center of the band behind the neck with both hands.

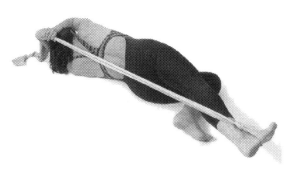

NOTE: If this exercise is too difficult for you, spread the center of the band over the upper shoulder and stabilize it with the upper hand.

EXERCISE: Bend your upper leg at the knee, using the knee as an axis or a hinge. Your lower leg will move behind the body while your thigh remains in place, so the hamstrings will be worked. Be sure your leg stays parallel to the floor as you bend and straighten it from the knee.

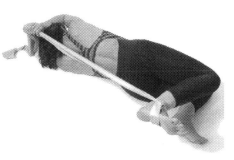

VI. POSTERIOR: THE JUNGLE CAT

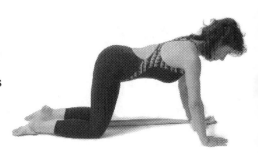

POSITION: Place your body in the all fours position. Straighten your back to create a 90° angle from your arms to your torso and from your thighs to your torso. Your abdominal muscles should support your lower back.

BAND: Place both ends of the band on the arch of your R foot. Stretch it underneath your body, holding the center of it with your L hand.

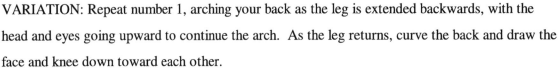

EXERCISE:

1. (a) Lengthen your R leg behind you by sliding the toes and the top of your foot on the floor, stretching the top of your quadriceps (front of thigh).

(b) Return to the original position.

VARIATION: Repeat number 1, arching your back as the leg is extended backwards, with the head and eyes going upward to continue the arch. As the leg returns, curve the back and draw the face and knee down toward each other.

2. Lengthen your R leg behind you by sliding it on the floor; then lift it to the height of your back. Return to the original position.

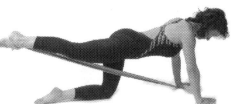

3. (a) Slide the R leg back, as in number 1.

(b) Continue to move it back even further, as if someone is pulling it.

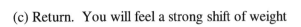

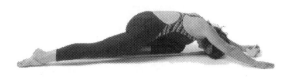

(c) Return. You will feel a strong shift of weight

backward on your hands so allow the back to move with the leg and keep the elbows slightly bent. The chin will drop down to the chest as your weight pulls back, and your head will look up on a diagonal when your weight goes forward again.

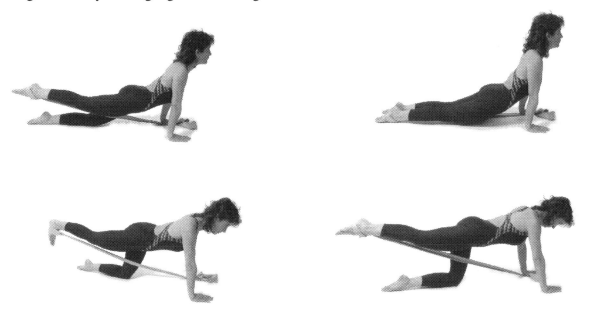

4. (a) Same as number 3. Extended the leg up at as high as your back.

  (b) Flex the foot as your leg moves outward and point it as it returns.

5. BEGINNING:

  (a) Slide the R foot on the floor behind you as in number 1.

  (b) Straighten the knee as you slide it to the side to a comfortable extension. The big toe will remain on the floor.

  (c) Slide it again behind you.

  (d) Return to the original position.

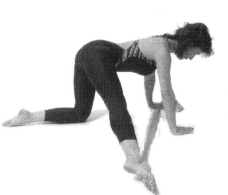

ADVANCED: Repeat number 5 with the leg at the height of your back.

6. BEGINNING:

(a) From the all fours position, lift your R leg in the air to the side while it is bent at the knee.

(b)Lower it to the floor.

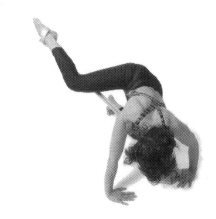

ADVANCED:

(a) Slide your R leg out to the side and straighten the leg, the big toe still on the floor.

(b) Lift your leg to the side as high in the air as it is comfortable, then lower it again to the floor.

(c) Repeat the leg lifts a certain number of times, whatever is appropriate for you.

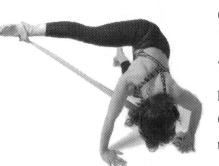

(d) Return the R leg to the starting position.

Keep both shoulders working evenly.

7. (a) Repeat number 1, straightening and lifting your R leg behind in parallel position. Lift as high as it is comfortable for you.

(b) Arch your back. Your head and eyes will look upward to continue the arch.

(c) Bring your R leg back in and underneath your body, curving the back and drawing the R knee and head toward each other.

(d) Repeat this exercise in turnout position.

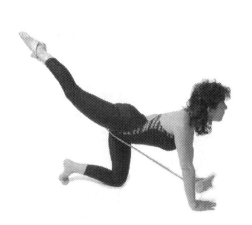

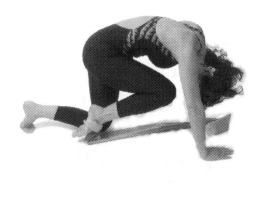

8. For the steps in this exercise, you may either move the band to the outside of your thigh or hold the center of the band with the same hand as the working leg.

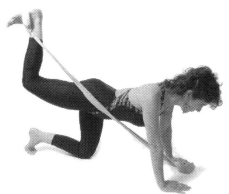

(a) Raise the R leg behind you to the height of your back, keeping your leg in a parallel position.

(b) Bend the R knee to create a 90° angle from your lower leg to thigh.

(c) Flex your R foot, so the sole will be facing the ceiling.

(d) Slowly lift the sole of your R foot toward the ceiling.

(d) Lower it until the thigh is even with the back.

(e) Bend the knee at 90° again. Make sure the knee of your R leg stays abducted toward the midline of your body. (Your knee and hip should be aligned with each other.)

NOTE: The abdominal muscles must remain contracted throughout the whole exercise, so it will support your lower back. Keep your rib cage closed like an umbrella, and bend your elbows slightly. Do not allow your weight to shift to the opposite hand when working with the leg to the side.

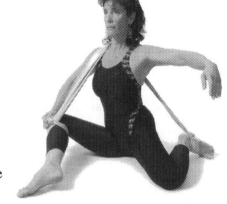

POSITION: Sit in fourth position, so your L leg is bent in front of your body and your R leg is bent behind you. This will create an open square between the inner sides of your R and L thighs. Your R knee should be behind you as much as it is comfortable. One of your hands will rest on the foot of your forward leg, and the other one will either be on the knee of your forward leg or beside it on the ground. Make sure your back is supported in the most erect position possible.

NOTE: Begin each exercise with your R leg rotated inward, so that the foot is lifted into the air while the thigh remains on the ground.

BAND: Attach the end of the band to your pointed R foot. Have the band come diagonally across the back and over the L shoulder. Wrap it once or twice over your L knee to stabilize the band.

EXERCISE:

1. Lower your R foot toward the floor, using your R knee as an axis. Allow your pelvis to rotate slightly backward as your foot presses down to the floor and rotate forward as your foot lifts up again.

2. Repeat number 1, except the movement of the leg and hip will be isolated. Do a smaller movement with the leg if you need to, as long as your hip remains fixated where it is as your R leg lifts up.

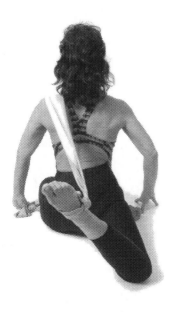

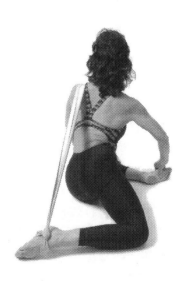

3. Straighten your R leg directly behind you. Extend it in an elongated line position aligned behind the R side of your back. As your foot reaches the floor, your knee will lift off the floor. As you return from that line, allow your R knee to come softly to the floor. Use your bent R knee as an axis to bend the lower leg back to the beginning position. For the transition in between the two sides, extend your lower R leg behind you in a straight line. Let the knee drop gently down on the floor. Rotate your R hip out to let the R knee come up toward the ceiling, and use your hands behind you for support. This will rotate your body halfway to the side. Round your back and rest in this position as long as needed, and then change the end of the band to the other foot. Rotate another quarter of a turn to the R side, and you will end up in the same position you started in, only facing the opposite direction. (Your R leg is now in front.) Now, you are ready to do the other side.

NOTE: In each stage of the exercise, try to bring your knee back a little further behind you.

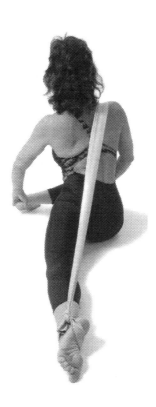

VIII. STRENGTHENING THE ADDUCTORS

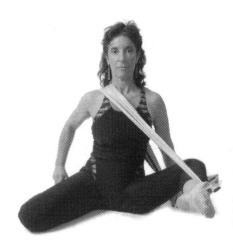

POSITION: Sit in fourth position with your R leg forward and your L leg behind.

BAND: Attach one end to the pointed R foot. Then, stretch the other end over the L shoulder, and hold in the L hand on the floor directly behind you. Be sure the band is taut enough to challenge you.

EXERCISE:

1. (a) Lift your R leg in an wide angle (slightly bent at the knee).

   (b) Shorten the band.

   (c) Slowly, lower your R leg down toward the floor.

NOTE:

1. (a) Try to keep your ankle and knee on the same level, parallel to the floor.

   (b) Do not allow your torso to sink down into the pelvis to achieve more height.

2. (a) Lift the front leg as in number 1.

   (b) Extend the leg forward into the ballet position developpe' devant.

   (c) Work very slowly and concentrate on keeping the heel up and leg turned out.

   (d) Bring the leg back to the bent angle with the same control.

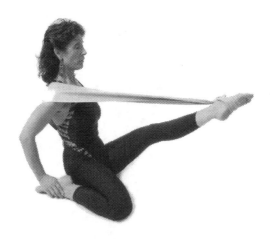

IX. THE PENDULUM

POSITION: Lie on your back. Your R leg is bent, so that the sole of the foot is flat on the floor, and the L knee is pointing up toward the ceiling. Bend the L leg and raise it up to your body, toward your chest; allow your L leg to open on a diagonal to the left side while still keeping the knee bent at the same angle.
BAND: Attach the end of the band to your pointed L foot and hold in your R hand.

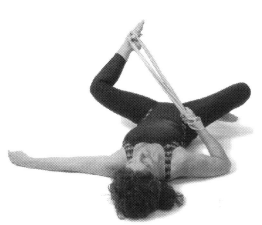

EXERCISE:

1. Keep both sides of the pelvis on the floor.

2. Using your knee as an axis, lower the L foot and lower leg down to the floor underneath you by rotating the thigh inwardly from the hip joint.

3. Return the L leg to beginning position.

 NOTE: As your lower leg rotates down, your L knee does not change the height you set at the beginning.

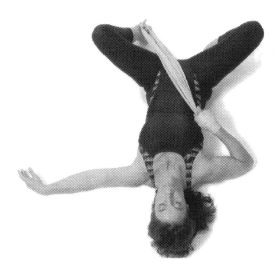

X. LEG ADDUCTORS

POSITION: Lie on your back. Bend your knees, drawing them up to your chest. Then, keeping your knees bent, open your legs wide.

BAND: Attach the ends of the band to each foot and hold the band with both hands at the center of the chest (sternum) at a point on the band that will provide you with the appropriate amount of resistance.

EXERCISE:

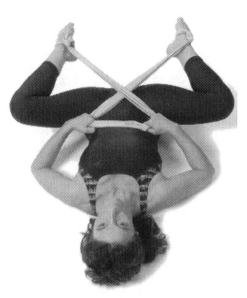

1. Leave the thighs and knees where they are. Open the lower part of both legs to make a straight line from the hips to the toes, creating a "V" with your legs. The pelvis will lift slightly off the ground as you move. Do the desired repetitions and return to the beginning position.

2. Repeat number 1, with the pelvis remaining on the ground.

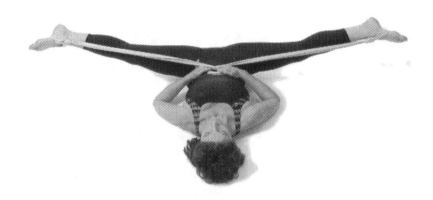

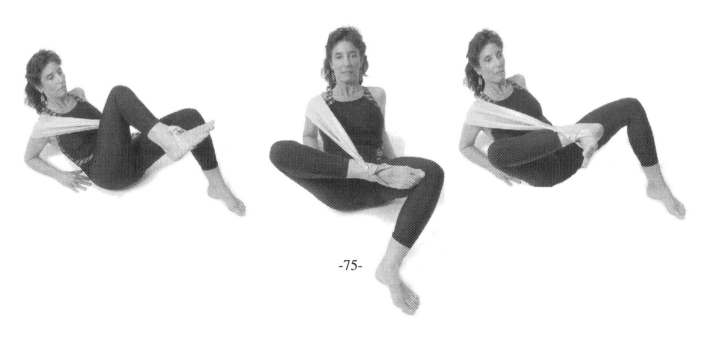

XI. THE INFINITY SYMBOL: ∞

NOTE: The following exercise is based on the Proprioceptive Neurological Facilitation (PNF) in physical therapy. It was developed by the neuro-physiologist Kabat, who believed that diagonal and spiral paths are inherent in the organization structure of muscular architecture and use.

POSITION: Sit down. Bend both knees, so the soles of the feet are flat on the floor. Point the knees toward the ceiling. Lean slightly backward, supporting your body weight behind you with your forearms on the floor. Both your elbows should be bent. Keep the torso elevated; do not let your shoulders shrug up or the body relax and slump down.

BAND: Attach one end of the band to your R foot. Stretch the remainder of the band across the torso, wrap once around the L hand, and hold to the floor to stabilize it.

EXERCISE:

1. With both hips on the floor, extend the R leg 45 to the side and diagonally upward. The band is stretched as the leg is extended and slackens as the knee bends. Think of tracing a horizontal figure eight (the symbol for infinity ∞) between the stationary knee and the diagonal, leading with the the big toe. Both hips will stay on the floor throughout the entire exercise, but you may move the upper body and head with the movement.

2. Repeat number 1, tracing the figure eight by leading with the little toe toward the knee and out to the diagonal, instead of the big toe.

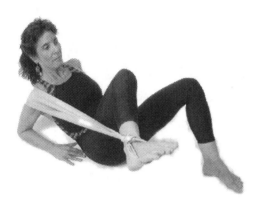
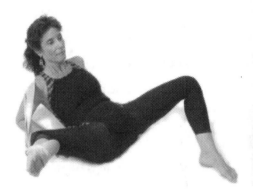

XII. ANTI GRAVITY FOOT WORK.

POSITION: Lie on your back with your legs straight up in the air at a 90° angle--you may use a wall, if needed. Your legs should not lean forward toward the face.
BAND: Place the ends of the band on the feet, crossed in front of the shins and held at center with hands. The elbows are bent and wide apart, pulling the band towards the floor.

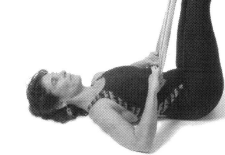

EXERCISE:

1. (a) Turn your legs outward at the hip joint, so
the feet are in a turned out first position--the
heels are together, and the toes are turned away
from each other.

(b) Point the feet as you bend both knees in a demi-plie'

(c) Stay in plie' while you flex both feet; then repeat for as many
repetitions as you need to do.

VARIATION:

1.Straighten the legs. Alternate the action of the feet: as the
R foot flexes; the L will point, etc.

2. Circle one foot at a time in a slow, full, outward circle;
first the L foot, then the R foot. Circle both feet outward at   the
same time.

3. Repeat number 2, except the circle will be inward instead of outward.

4 (a) Circle your foot inward while you circle your L foot outward.

(b) Repeat, changing feet.

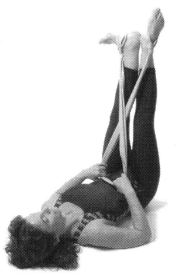

XIII. CALF AND FOOT: REVVING THE ACCELERATOR

(WORKING AGAINST A CHAIR)

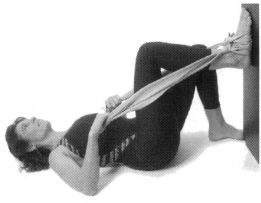

POSITION: Lie on your back with your R leg resting on the seat of a chair and the sole of your R foot against the chair back. Anchor the chair against a wall to keep it steady as you work. NOTE: If you do not have a chair of the right height for you, you may also do this entire exercise section lying on your back in front of a wall, with your R knee bent at a 90° angle (as if you were resting it on a chair), and the sole of your R foot flattened against the wall.

BAND: Place both ends of the band across the metatarsal of the sole of the R foot. Run the band along both sides of the R calf.

BEGINNING: Hold one strand of the band in the right hand at the R side of your calf; hold the other strand of the band in the left hand at the L side of your calf.

ADVANCED: Run both strands of the band along the inside of your R leg. Use your R hand to hold the center of the band. Bend your elbows and bring your R fist to the R shoulder. Your L hand will help to stabilize the band, just below the R hand.

EXERCISE: 1. Raise your heel away from the chair back to a position where your toes are touching and are flat on the chair, the rest of the foot is elevated away from the chair. Make sure all five toes are still against the back of the chair. Return slowly.

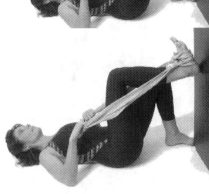

ADVANCED: Position your R foot higher on the chair or wall and repeat the exercise.

2. Extend the toes to full-point, so that your big toe is hardly touching the chair.

3. Slowly, go through the position where your toes are resting on the chair. Flatten the sole of the foot to the chair again.

4. Fixate the heel against the chair and allow the toes and the center of the foot to flex.

5. Return to starting position.

1.

To be where there is no movement and no touch is a horrifying thought.

2

Movement is everywhere. It is always happening, whether we think about it or not. Try this: Stand still for a minute and pay attention. There is so much that goes on. Were you even aware of it? For example, can you sense the tendons running along each side of your ankle? There are many indistinguishable readjustments that happen every moment in order to support your body and stabilize your balance.

3

Balance is a very significant word for me. This is illustrated in my five- year-old daughter's first visit to the dentist. Remembering my experiences, I knew a child's first trip to the dentist requires psychological preparation. The dentist was kind. At the outset, he allowed her to handle some of his instruments, the small mirrors, the air jet and water syringe. Furthermore, he allowed her, as part of his philosophy, to establish the tempo for all that was about to happen to her. While appreciating her enjoyment, the dentist said, "What a bright -eyed little girl you have." I replied, "Is that unusual?" "Oh yes," he said, "so many of them have eyes of blah." "Blah," I asked? "Eyes like glass," he continued. "Comes from hours and hours of watching TV." As you can see balance is a very important word for me.

4

When teaching about the torso muscle initiating movement or the idea of crossing the band--with the band from the right foot held in the left hand and vice versa, I imagine the shape of a building's scaffold, with the beams crossed in an "x" shape to give it support and strength.

#5

We are bombarded with nutritional information from nutritionists, books, and television telling us we must have a balanced diet. You must have the proper amount of protein, starch, fat, milk, fruits, vegetables, etc. each day. Each authority sets forth his or her own set of measures. This confused me. In addition, I was forever getting hung up on "Yes, but...." A case in point, a banana is a fruit, but it is also starch, so where do I categorize it? In the end, I have to find my own "balance.". To me, balance means stay simple. Separate foods. For example, after a lunch made of peanut butter (protein) on whole grain bread (starch)I feel tired. On the other hand, protein by itself in one meal and starch in the next feel easier on my digestive system. For me, simplicity and separation is proper balance. Each person must find his or her own balance.

6

Each one of us has a different hand signature and a specific, unique handwriting. What exactly makes this so? Some psychology experts say that there are personality traits which will explain this phenomenon, but physiologically, we each differ in now we hold our pen, how we move our fingers to create the letter shape, and in the amount of pressure that our pen puts ink on the paper.

7

Have you ever stepped off of a ship onto solid ground or a moving train while it is slowing down ? Remember how the movement of the ship and feeling of inner rocking still stayed with you for hours? I enjoy that unusual inner space.

8

As a teacher, I find it is often difficult to know how much of what I teach is actually being absorbed by my students. One year, at the end of the semester, I asked my students in the dance department at the University of South Florida to come up with one thing they learned about themselves from taking my class.

I remember one dancer, in particular, who brought some of her own shoes for this assignment as a kind of "show-and-tell" demonstration. First, she showed the class a pair of flat-heeled shoes which had a clear imprint of her foot on the front part of the inner soles. She made the connection between her posture and the way her weight was distributed on her feet. There was also a pair of yellow shoes with very high heels. She used these shoes of hers to explain how the height of the heel could account for the tightness and shortness of her hamstring muscles. I went home smiling that day.

9

Have you ever seen those beautiful arches in the ceilings of the ancient churches in Europe or the arches of the Roman aqueduct? Your bones have the same arched inner structure. Taking that thought one step further, stand. Put your feet together side by side. Look down at them. Can you see the arches of your feet creating a dome shape? Can you see the strength and support that is carried up your legs and into your pelvic floor? Can you see the benefit of this support?

#10

    As a child, do you remember playing with the toy made from a coiled wire spring--a Slinky? Think of how fluidly it moved when you pushed it gently from the top of the stairs and it would begin to ripple down the steps, turning end over end, until it reached the bottom. Remember how it locked when you held it from the top ring and let it spiral down toward the floor. We can apply the spiral principle of the Slinky to stand up with a more efficient se of energy. The next time you get up from a chair, try to imitate that same spiral pattern. Place one foot slightly in front of the other, then think of rotating your hip and shifting your weight over your feet as you rise. Do you feel the ease of doing this as opposed to trying to just "power" your way to a standing position? Try the same thing from sitting on the floor in a crossed-legged position, basically leaving the feet in the same place where they are at the start. For example, if your right foot is in front as you sit, you will cross the right foot over the left knee. Begin to rotate the hip and torso to the left while pushing with the left hand into the floor behind you. Turn the head and eyes upward to the left to precede the body. Keep a low center of gravity to hold your balance. By the time you have rotated into a standing position, you will have made a complete half-turn to face the opposite direction.

#11

  Have you ever seen those beautiful arches in the ceilings of the ancient churches in Europe or the arches of the roman aqueduct? Your bones have the same arched inner structure. Taking that thought one step further; stand, put your feet together, side by side. Look down at them. Can you see the arches of your feet creating a dome shape? Can you visualize the strength and support that is carried up your legs and into your pelvic floor? Can you see the benefit of this support?

#12

The nervous system is like a governor. In other words, it should be a precise perception of the attention and intention we put into the body. If we find a way to reeducate our bodies to perform better quality movement, that means, we have to uncover stages in our developmental progress that are unfinished. For example relearn how to crawl with opposition of right leg with left arm. Doing this will correct our difficulties originating at that time of development. Your nervous system, in conjunction with your brain, has the extraordinary power to improve, heal, and allow choices of movement in the body.

#13

I remember one Tuesday afternoon that I and off from the army camp. I rushed to the city to pamper myself, so I could feel a little feminine again. By the time it was dark, I saw an unclear image of a person moving, walking a couple of blocks in front of me. I looked again, and it suddenly hit me. I thought to myself, "Oh yeah, that's my mom!" I went forward to greet her. I had not seen her for a month. From that distance, in the light, it would seem to be impossible to tell for sure who it was. So how did I know? The first thing I recognized was her walk. I saw her familiar head swing, and the movement of her shoulders up and down, forward and back. You may have had the same experience as well, knowing who someone was simply because the way they walk. Perhaps you did not break it down into its elements at the time, but somehow, you just knew. We all make unconscious choice of how to use our body when we walk. What is your movement (or lack of movement) in the shoulders when you lift the opposite hip? Do you move your pelvis, or do you swing from your legs down? Does your shoulders move up and down forward and back with each stance? How much do your knees bend?

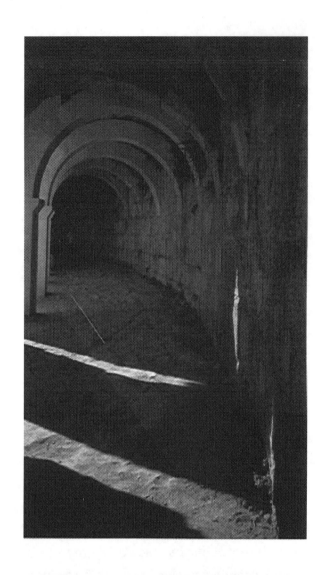

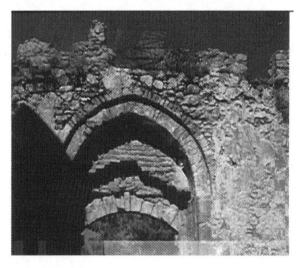

Part 3:

UPPER BODY

"WHEN HE IS BORN, MAN IS SOFT AND WEAK; IN DEATH HE BECOMES STIFF AND HARD. THE TEN THOUSAND THINGS, AND ALL PLANTS AND TREES WHILE THEY ARE ALIVE ARE SUPPLE AND SOFT, BUT WHEN THEY ARE DEAD THEY ARE BRITTLE AND DRY. TRULY, WHAT IS STIFF AND HARD IS A 'COMPANION OF DEATH', WHAT IS SOFT AND YIELDING IS A 'COMPANION OF LIFE.'"

LAO TZU

MUSCLES OF THE SHOULDER GIRDLE

1. Trapezius

2. Levator scapula

3. Rhomboideus

4. Serratus anterior

5. Pectoralis minor

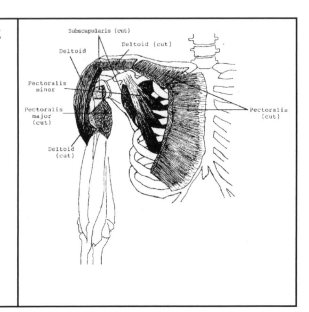

MUSCLES OF THE SHOULDER JOINT

1. Deltoideus

2. Supraspinatus

3. Infraspinatus

4. Subscapularis

5. Teres major

6. Latissimus dorsi

7. Pectoralis major

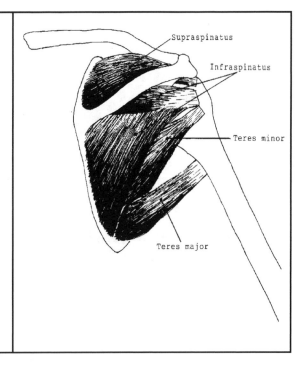

MUSCLES OF THE ARM

1. Biceps brachii
2. Brachialis
3. Brachioradialis
4. Triceps
5. Pronator teres

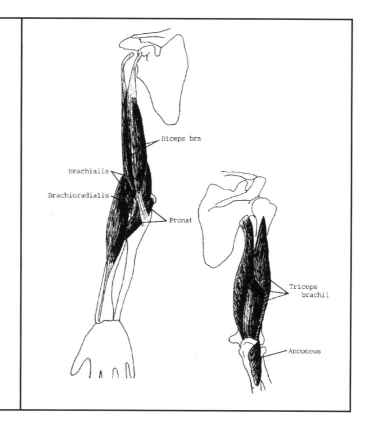

MUSCLES OF THE LATERAL TORSO

1. Serratus anterior
2. Quadratus lumboum
3. Obliquus externus
4. Obliquus internus abdominalis
5. Intercostal internal
6. Intercostal externalI.

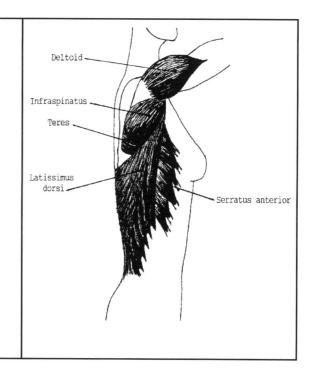

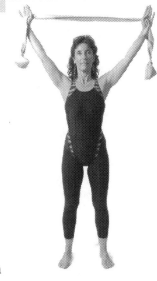

NOTE: Most of the exercises in this section can be done in either a sitting or in a standing position unless it is otherwise specified.

POSITION: Hold the arms over the head at a distance that is a little wider than shoulder width apart. Slightly bend the elbows.

Rotate backward to keep them from locking.

BAND: Hold the band with both hands over the head.

EXERCISES: NOTE: To achieve the maximum results for the arm and back muscles, do each exercise once all the way through with the arm rotated out (palm and fingers facing up) and once with the arm rotated in (palm and fingers facing down).

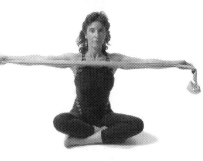

1. Exhale while slowly stretching the band directly to each side until the hands are at shoulder height. The band will be stretched onto your shoulders, just behind your head.

2. Repeat number 1, stretching the band in front of the face as you pull your arms to the sides.

3. (a) Hold the band down in front of your body.

   (b) Extend both arms directly to each side, moving them upward until they are at shoulder height.

NOTE: Do this exercise once holding the band with the palms facing up and once with the palms facing down.

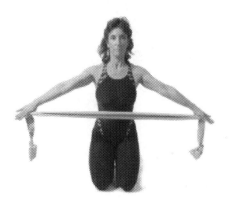

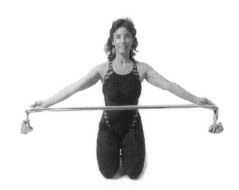

4. Repeat number 3, holding the band behind the body as you raise your arms instead of in front of it.

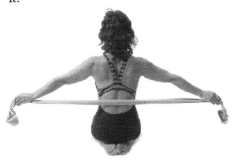 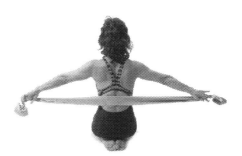

5. (a) Hold the band in both hands.

(b) Extend your arms directly forward.

(c) Open your arms to each side, keeping the same relationship between the arms and the body.
NOTE: Do not let the shoulder blades "pinch" together; instead, try to widen the back by thinking of your shoulder blades staying as far away from your spine as possible.

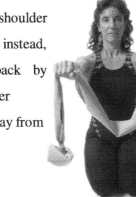 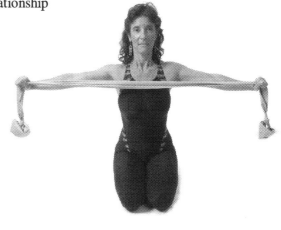

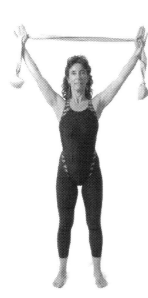

6. ROTATION: (a) Stand with the legs   parallel, about hip width apart. The arms will hold the band above the head at about shoulder width.

(b) Rotate the upper body from the waist to face the L side; the hips remain facing forward. While in this position, stretch the band with both arms going directly to each side, to about the height of your shoulders, then continue bringing the arms down in front of the L thigh.

(c) Rotate the upper body from the waist to the R side, hips still facing forward. Reverse the arm movement that you did while facing the other direction--raise both arms directly to each side (the band stretching the most when they reach shoulder level), and continue until the arms are overhead as far apart as your shoulders. Rotate the torso to face directly forward, as in the beginning of this exercise.

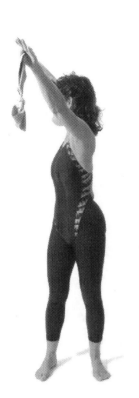 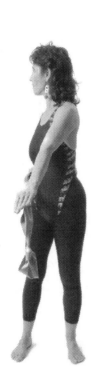 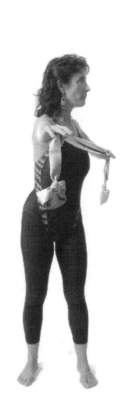 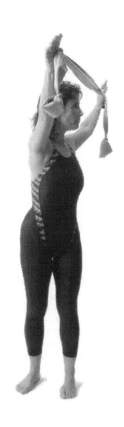

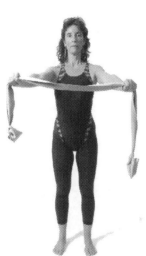

VARIATIONS: In order to work the biceps, do the following three exercises holding the band with your palms up; hold your palms down if you wish to work the triceps. Begin each variation with both arms extended directly forward, as in number 5.

(a) Open the R arm to an upward diagonal and the L arm to a downward diagonal, both arms working at the same time.

(b) Keep the L arm in original position, directly forward. Isolate the R arm by lowering it down in a diagonal. This exercise will specifically work the triceps.)

(c) Keep the L arm in original position, directly forward. Isolate the R arm by raising it up in a diagonal. (This exercise will specifically work the biceps.)

8. ABDUCTION (in the frontal plane):

(a) Place one end of the band on the R foot.

(b) Step forward slightly with the R foot, holding the band in the R hand by your side at a point on the band which is comfortable for you.

(c) Lengthen the band upwards, directly to the R side, as far as shoulder height.

NOTE: If this version is too difficult for you, the position for this exercise can be modified. From the R foot, the band is stretched up behind you, over the R elbow, and over the R shoulder. The R hand will hold the band in front of the chest. You can now push the band out to the side with your elbow instead of the whole arm. You will find this to be easier since the lever (your arm) is half the length as it was before.

9. FLEXION: Repeat number 7, raising the R arm directly in front of you to shoulder height, instead of to the side. This will contract your pectoralis muscle.

10. HORIZONTAL ABDUCTION/ADDUCTION: Begin the exercise as in number 7. Next, move your R arm (with elbow straightened but not locked) from the side of the body to directly forward, then back again. Keep the same distance between the arm and body as you move.

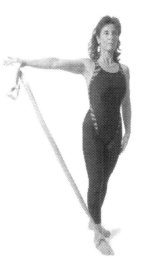

II   CHEST PRESS

POSITION: Stand with the upper arms at the sides of the body; bend the elbows at a 90° angle, parallel to the floor.

BAND: Run the band across the scapulas (shoulder blades) and under the armpits. Hold the band in each hand at a place on the band that will provide you with the appropriate amount of resistance

EXERCISES:

1. (a) Press the arms and hands directly forward so the arms are extended in front of you.

(b) Return to the beginning position.

(c) Try to press the arms forward an inch higher each time.

(d) Once you work up to the highest diagonal, hold your arms out in the extended position, then raise and lower your arms so your shoulder joint acts as a hinge. Be sure to keep the shoulder blades depressed.

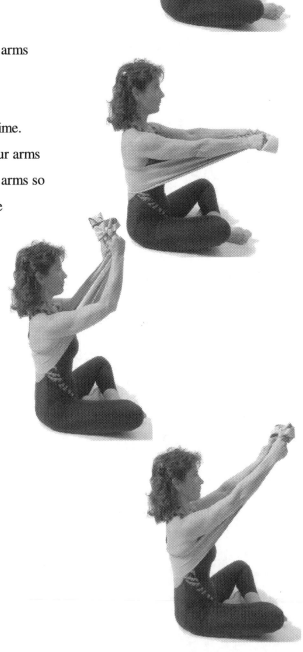

2. (a) Same beginning position.

(b) Keeping the elbows in the same 90 degree relationship, raise the arms by pushing the elbows away from the body.

NOTE: At completion, the upper arms should be at shoulder height (parallel to the floor), and the lower arms should be perpendicular to them.

III. BICEPS

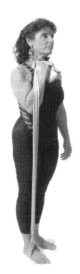

POSITION: Stand with the R foot slightly ahead of the L. Brace the R upper arm against the body and bend the lower arm at a 90○ angle.

BAND: Wrap both ends over the R foot. Hold the center in the R hand with the palm facing up.

EXERCISE:

1. Keeping the R elbow held against the body, bring the R palm, wrist, and forearm up, toward the R shoulder.

2. Slowly return to starting position.

Note: Do not bend your wrist while doing the exercise.

IV. TRICEPS

POSITION: Stand. Bend the R arm close to your side, so that your R hand is near the R shoulder. Bend the L arm, and hold in front of your chest.

BAND: Hold both ends of the band in your L hand, which will remain stationary throughout the exercise. With your R hand, hold the doubled band at a point that will provide you with the appropriate amount of resistance.

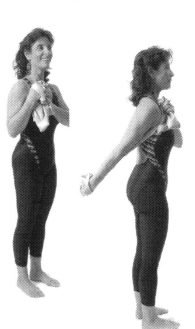

EXERCISE:

1. Extend the right hand and arm down toward the right side of the body.

2. Slightly behind it, using the R elbow as an axis.

3. Return slowly to starting position.

Variation - hold the band behind the head lengthening the hand and the forearm above the head

V. THE SHAWL

POSITION: Sit comfortably, crossed legged in front of you. Bend your arms at the elbows and hold your hands at a small distance in front of your chest. Lift the elbows to each side and turn your hands slightly outward, so the backs of your hands are facing toward you. (This position will be clearer to you as you stretch the band into the "shawl position," which is described below.)

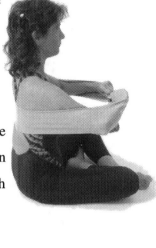

BAND: For the "shawl position," place the center of the band is on your spine. The rest of the band is spread over your shoulder blades (which are kept wide open), on top of the shoulders, down each arm, and over each elbow. Hold the band with each hand (palms turned out) at a point which is comfortable for you.

EXERCISES:

1. (a) Using the elbow as an axis and keeping both elbows lifted, open and extend the hands and forearms out to the side.

    (b) Return slowly.

2. Repeat number 1 with the palms and fingers turned in.

3. Same starting position.

(a) Extend the arms directly forward without locking the elbows.

(b) Return slowly.

4. Repeat number 3 with the palms and fingers turned in.

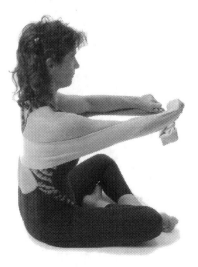

VI. SHAWL VARIATION

POSITION: Sit in a wide second position on the floor. Point your knees up to the ceiling.

BAND: Attach each end of the band to each foot with the center of the band behind the back, passing underneath the scapula. Stretch the band above the elbows, which are bent slightly toward the back. Hold the band with each hand to stabilize it.

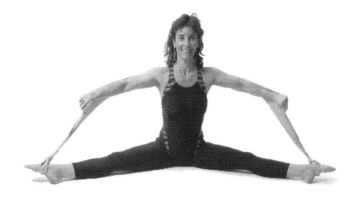

EXERCISE:

1. Contract your abdominal muscles, letting your head and spine curve over (as if you were looking at your belly button)and allow your pelvis to roll backward. Make sure you lift your elbows and widen your back.

2. Lengthen your arms out toward your feet.

3. Return by lifting the pelvis back to erect position, rolling the spine up, and bending the elbows.

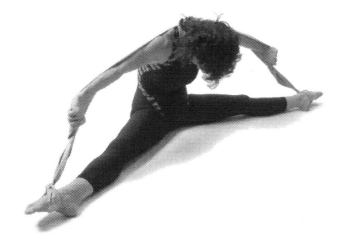

VII. CRESCENT BEND

POSITION: Straighten both your arms overhead at a distance that is a little wider than shoulder width. Have the legs parallel, about hip width apart.

NOTE: You will be lying in this position on the floor in exercise number 1. All other exercises will be done in a standing position.

BAND: Hold the band stretched in each hand, the ends of the band hanging down on each side of your arms.

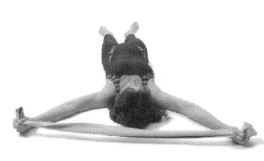

EXERCISES:

1. Lay on the floor.

(a) Keep the L arm stationary. Your R arm will pull the band down to the R side as the body curves into a crescent shape. Think of bending vertebra by vertebra, all the way down to the pelvis, without actually shifting the pelvis from center.

(b) Slowly return to the starting position by bringing the R arm to the L arm, and leading with the L ribs.

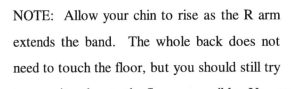

NOTE: Allow your chin to rise as the R arm extends the band. The whole back does not need to touch the floor, but you should still try to press it as low to the floor as possible. You may bend your knees if they feel overly stressed. Do not release your abdominal muscles or rib cage.

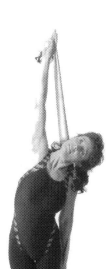

2. Repeat number 1 while standing in parallel first position.

3. Repeat number 2. Having bent your torso over to the R side, you will not initiate the rolling up from the L ribs; instead, you will reach the L arm up toward the ceiling. Create the feeling of the L arm pulling you up to the starting position.

4. Repeat number 2, bending to the side with your arms maintaining their same distance to each other and to your head. Then, instead of initiating the rolling up from the ribs or the arm, think of lifting the whole torso up as a single unit.

NOTE: Do not allow your torso to tilt forward as you bend to the side; keep your body facing directly to the front. Lengthen the arms outward, press down the scapulas, and fixate your torso in that position. Keep your rib cage in.

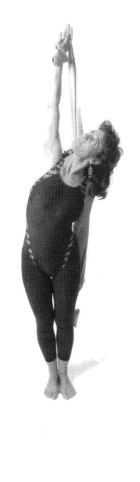

Variations:

A. Have your head face down, or up to work different muscle groups in your neck & shoulder.

B. Bend your knees to increase the difficulty.

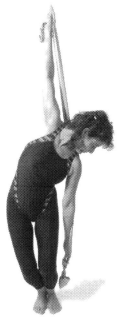

VIII. HALF-MOON TWIST

POSITION: Stand in a parallel first position. Slightly bend the knees , and keep the arms overhead about shoulder width apart.

BAND: Hold the band over your head with both hands.

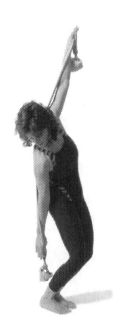

EXERCISE:

1. Stretch your torso and upper body laterally to the L side.

2. While you are bending, stretch both arms to each side until they are at shoulder level. (Place the band behind the head so that it is almost resting on the shoulders).

3. Bend as far over to the side as you can without allowing the R hip to shift out of alignment and keep the hips centered.

4. While you are still bent over to the side, rotate the torso from the waist one quarter of a turn to the L side, as if you are trying to look at the floor.

5. Rotate back again to the lateral bend to the side, facing forward.

6. Slowly straighten the body back to the original upright position by initiating the torso lift from the upper arm.

7. Roll the body up one vertebra at a time. The abdominal muscles Should support the back muscles.

Variation -The same exercise with the knees bent

IX. LATERALS

POSITION: Sit with the legs in a wide second position (straddle split), as far to each side as comfortable. The torso is upright and the arms are held over the head, shoulder width apart.

BAND: Hold the band in both hands comfortably, neither stretched nor loose.

EXERCISES:

1. (a) Isolate the R arm, and open it to the R side. (b) Return.

2. (a) Shift the body to the R side by leading with the R ribs. The R arm will reach out and up on a diagonal, but only to the point where you are still sitting on both hips; leave the L arm where it is.

    (b) Return to starting position.

3. (a) Curve your upper body over to the R side, initiating the movement from the head.

(b) Stretch each side of the band to shoulder level as you bend; the R arm will open downward, and the L arm will stretch upward.

(c) Return to starting position.

4. (a) Bend the body laterally as in number 3.

    (b) At the depth of your bend, rotate the torso down to face the leg.

    (c) Use your opposite hip and abdominal muscles to turn the torso   back to the lateral bend.

    (d) Lift your torso to return to the upright position.

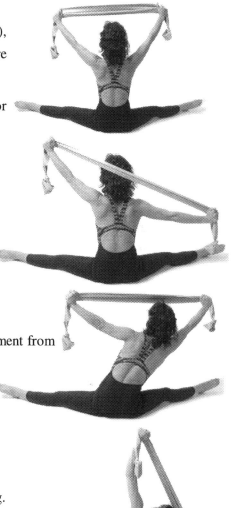

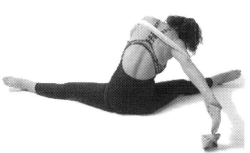

VARIATION: Repeat these exercises with your legs in different positions: a little less wide in your sitting second position, a parallel first position, or cross-legged.

-99-

X. ADVANCED LATERALS

POSITION: Sit with both legs wide in a second position, as far apart as possible. Keep the knees facing up toward the ceiling.

BAND: Place one end of the band is on the R foot. Hold the band at a point that will provide the right amount of resistance for you with your R hand, or for more of a workout, with your L hand.

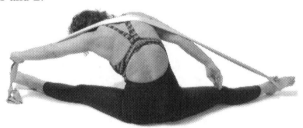

EXERCISES:

1. (a) Shift the body, so the torso and arm stretch up on a

   diagonal to the L side.

   (b) Hold this position for a few seconds.

   (c) Return.

2. (a) Bend your body laterally to the L side, so your face and body are forward.

   (b) At the depth of your bend, turn your face and body down as if you were looking at the L leg.

   (c) Use the right side of your hip and abdominal muscles to rotate the body back to the lateral bend.

   (d) Lift the body up to the starting position.

3. Create a smooth combination of numbers 1 and 2.

XI. HANDS OF THE CLOCK

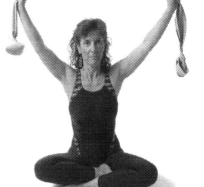

POSITION: Sit in any comfortable position on the floor or on the edge of a chair, making certain that both sides of your body remain equal.

BAND: Hold the band above your head slightly wider than shoulder width apart and a little behind the head, so the arms will act as an extension of the back. Keep your shoulder blades depressed as much as possible.

EXERCISE:

Note: For each exercise, your L arm will remain free.

1. " Lift your head" and neck, extending them, then create a big arch by moving your head toward your R arm, leading with the R ear. Note: Your nose will face **forward** during the entire exercise.

2. (a) Depress the R shoulder blade, and lift your R arm up toward your ear.

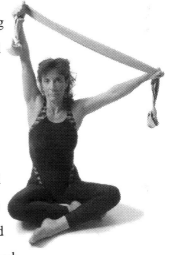

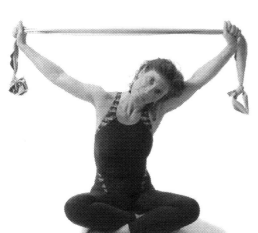

3. COMBINATION of number 1 and 2: The head will arch down to the R side. The R arm will lift, and both will meet at the center of the arch.

NOTE: Remember to-

Depress the shoulder blades each time you raise or lower your arms.

 Keep the eyes and nose focused forward.

 Do not protrude the ribs forward.

1

Losing weight--losing fat. We know by now our main goal for good health is to maintain a lean body. This does not necessarily mean losing weight, per se; it simply means that we should alter our fat-to-lean body ration, so the fat percentage is within a desirable range. It would be best to empty some of our fat cells and increase the muscle fibers. Even if the actual numbers on the scale do not change that much, our overall appearance will improve. We also know in order to achieve this goal, we should eat a balance of foods which are low in fat content, as well as doing physical activity which is at a low intensity (60-70%) for a relatively long duration (one hour) on a regular basis. Therefore, why is it hard for us to put this knowledge into practice? Why is it that every single time I pass by my bathroom scale I step on it, looking for the results with anticipation, just like I have been doing for the last twenty years? The answer is one word: habit. Think of the habits you have acquired over your lifetime. Can you come up with one of them that you would like to change?

2

There are many places where we can find movement if look for it. When I was a child, I remember seeing a photograph of oil on a small pool of water. It was a color photo, so I could see the wonderful colors swirling with the motion of the water. Another place where I remember seeing movement was in the multicolored specs of the terrazzo tiles on our bathroom floor. When I used my imagination, I saw connections between the different colored patterns, and I made the shapes into a story.

3

One of my favorite places of movement is the clouds. I used to walk home from school with my head back, gazing up at them, watching them sail past. They became animals, historic figures, or characters from mysterious stories, depending on how the wind blew them. Now, thirty years later, I still watch them when I lie back in my hammock or in the Jacuzzi. The movement up in the sky is still going on.

4

    During my last year of my army service, I was stationed at a remote little kibbutz out in the Israeli desert. It was really a very harsh transition when I decided to leave the kibbutz and move to the crowded city of Tel Aviv. Once I got there, I remember seeing people everywhere I looked. I developed a great fear of crowds because I was not used to so many people around me at one time. The main street in Tel Aviv, Dizingoff Street, was the busiest of all. It was also the street I had to walk through every day to get to my apartment. I tried to shield myself from my fear by concentrating on just a specific part of everyone around me. For example, as I passed through the street on any given day, I might see only eyes; on another day, it might be lips, or shoulder movements, or the tops of heads, and so on. I found that if only separated the people into smaller parts, then I could cope with them. This proved to be a very effective way to deal with a street pavement full of walking people.

5

    I had a dance student come to me one morning to talk. She told me about a disturbing incident she had experienced in the past and how it had affected her life, her dreams, and her relationships. Her nervous system was filled with emotion. Her cry carried through her whole body. All I could do for her at that moment was to put my hand firmly on her sternum to allow her to bring herself to awareness and to give her the time a space she needed. Dance and movement were her means of release and escape, but she could not pursue it until she worked out this other major issue. She dropped from the dance program, knowing that she could not truly do it well until she worked through her past and healed.

6

    Imagine having a high rise on the seashore. In the distance, you can see an open place. In that open space, your movement possibilities are endless. What would you choose to do?

7

Imagine taking a risk: Dance with your eyes closed, supporting the inner focus, diving into your own depth, finding you own body expressions (not just repeating movements you have already learned). Can you let your movement flow naturally, without projection, without interpretation, or without judgement? Can you trust yourself fully by stepping outside what you consider "safe"?   That is being authentic.

8

Awareness is one of the elements--along with physical and internal sensation, movement, thought and feelings--that makes up our self-image. Awareness is how we know what we know about ourselves. One exercise to increase our own awareness is by scanning the body. Lie down on the floor and imagine you are looking at yourself from the ceiling. Compare the two sides of your body. What do you see?   Now draw your attention inward. Try to sense the spaces between your body and the floor and the points at which your body weight creates pressure against the floor. Now pay attention to the inner sensations of your bone, muscles, fluids, and organs. This process takes time. It is an a internal "listening:" to master. Give yourself at least twenty to thirty minutes each time you do this exercise in order to develop your skills. Do not become discouraged and give up halfway through. Allow yourself the time you need to create a new relationship within yourself.

9

When the book was going through its final "winding-up" stages, with the photographs being organized and assigned to the correct pages, a tremendous source of movement forced us to sit up and take notice of it; it was Hurricane Andrew. Besides the danger and destruction, it was really fascinating to watch the hurricane from above--the spiral movement of the clouds circling on the outskirts of the storm, the short-lived peace in the eye. However, the beauty of it ends once you find that you are caught in its raging path.

10

Another way to relax those tired trapezius muscles on the days that you feel like Hercules with the whole world resting on your shoulders: Shrug your shoulders up toward your ears, and hold them there as tensely as you can. You should begin to get a warm, shivering sensation. Hold them there for a while; then simply let them drop to their normal position as you exhale. Although it seems that tensing the shoulder muscles will only make them feel worse, they actually will feel freer and more relaxed.

PART 4

WARM-UP CLOSURE

EVERY MAN IS THE BUILDER OF A TEMPLE, CALLED HIS BODY, TO THE GOD HE WORSHIPS, AFTER A STYLE PURELY HIS OWN, NOR CAN HE GET OFF BY HAMMERING MARBLE INSTEAD. WE ARE ALL SCULPTORS AND PAINTERS, AND OUR MATERIAL IS OUR OWN FLESH AND BLOOD AND BONES. ANY NOBLENESS BEGINS AT ONCE TO REFINE A MAN'S FEATURES, ANY MEANNESS WITH SENSUALITY TO IMBRUTE THEM.

HENRY DAVID THOREAU

Walden and Other Writings Page 199,

Editor Brook Atkinson, 1937, & 1950

Random House Inc, The Modern Library N.Y.

MUSCLES OF THE POSTERIOR BACK

1. Erector spinae	9. Iliocostalis dorsi	15. Suboccipital
2. Spinalis dorsi	10. Iliocostalis cervicis	16. Serratus superior
3. Spinalis cervicis	11. Splenius capitis	17. Serratus inferior
4. Spinalis capitis	12. Splenius cervicis	18. Interspinales of the entire spinal column
5. Longissimus dorsi	13. Rotators of the entire spinal column	
6. Longissimus cervicis		19. Intertransversalis of the entire spinal column
7. Longissimus capitis	14. Multifidus of the entire spinal column	
8. Iliocostalis lumborum		

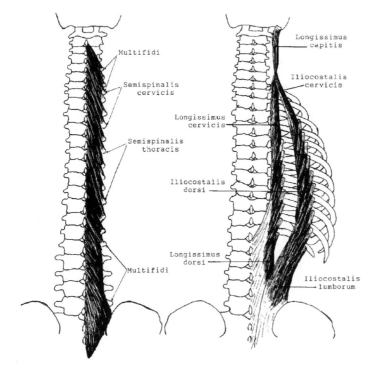

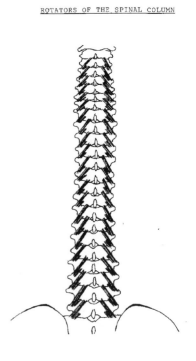

ROTATORS OF THE SPINAL COLUMN

MUSCLES OF THE ANTERIOR TORSO

1. Rectus abdominalis
2. Obliquus externus abdominalis
3. Obliquus internus abdominalis

4. Transversus abdominalis
5. Intercostal external
6. Intercostal internal

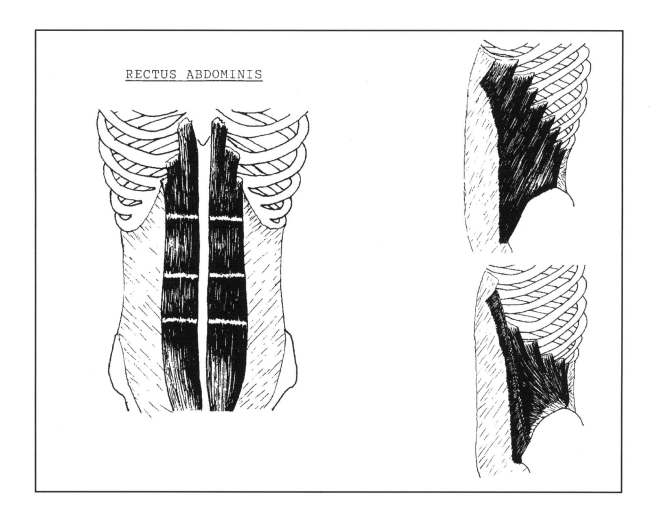

RECTUS ABDOMINIS

MUSCLES OF THE HEAD AND NECK

1. Longus colli	8. Scalenus medius
2. Longus capitis	9. Scalenus posterior
3. Rectus capitis anterior	10. Splenius capitis
4. Rectus capitis lateralis	11. Splenius cervicis
5. Rectus capitis posterior major	12. Obliquus capitis inferior
6. Rectus capitis posterior minor	13. Obliquus superiorI
7. Scalenus anterior	

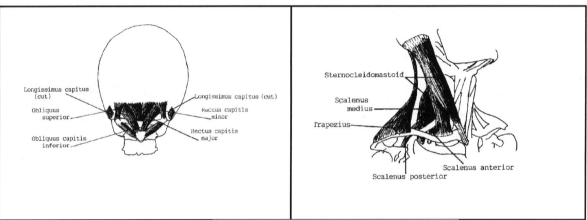

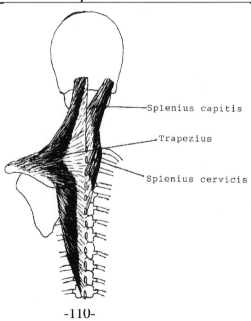

I THE BODY BUILDER STRETCH

POSITION: Lie on the floor on your back with your legs about hip width apart. Bend the legs, and point both knees up toward the ceiling. Place the soles of the feet flat on the floor.

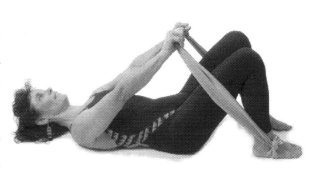

BAND: Place the ends of the band on each foot. Run the remainder of the band runs the outside of the ankle, and then hold in each hand. Hold both arms about chest width apart with the elbows straightened, but not hyper extended. Hold the band directly above your navel.

EXERCISES: 1.(a) Bring the arms directly overhead and down toward the floor as much as you can without arching the back.

(b) Return the arms slowly to beginning position again.

2. In this exercise, the L foot and R arm will work together.

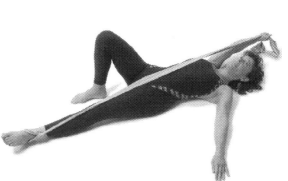

(a) Hold the band over your navel with the R hand alone. The L arm is on the floor at your side, with the palm facing down in order to stabilize yourself to keep balance.

(b) Extend the L foot 90° up toward the ceiling.

(c) Lower the straightened leg to the floor below you by pulling the leg out of the hip joint.

(d) At the same time, the R arm and the band will stretch overhead to the floor.

(e) Slowly, return to the beginning position by reversing the movements.

3. Repeat number 2, holding the band with the L hand. Instead of working in opposition, you will be working the same arm and leg.

4. In this exercise, both arms and both legs will be working together.

(a) Hold the band with both hands directly in front of you.

(b) Extend both legs straight up into the air. The arms will go to the floor overhead at the same time as the legs will go to the floor below you.

(c) Slowly, return to the beginning position by reversing the movements.

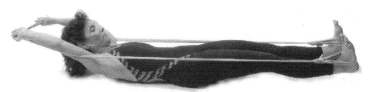

NOTE: As you become stronger, you will need less band length from your hands to your feet.

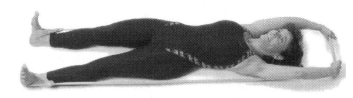

II. PRONE: THE ARCHER'S BOW

POSITION: Lie in a prone position (on your stomach) with your face down. Extend your arms overhead. Extend your legs below your body.

BAND: Attach one end of the band to the L foot. Hold the other end in the R hand at a point on the band which will give you the right amount of resistance.

EXERCISES:

1. (a) Simultaneously, lift the R arm and the L leg off the floor, lengthening the limbs from their joints before lifting them.

 (b) Return slowly to the floor again.

2. With the band stretched, isolate and work the R arm only.

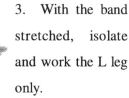

3. With the band stretched, isolate and work the L leg only.

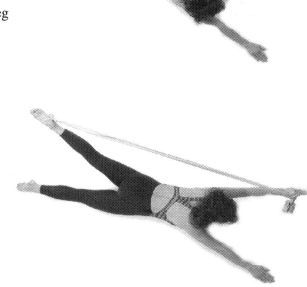

4. (a) Attach the ends of the band to the R leg and the R hand, so you are working the same side of the body.

 (b) Repeat numbers 1-3.

III. DEEP ROTATION OF THE BACK I (ADVANCED)

POSITION: Lie in a prone position (on your stomach) with your face down. Extend your arms overhead. Extend your legs below your body.

BAND: Attach one end of the band to the R foot. Run the remainder of the band along the R side of the back, over the R shoulder, and then hold it over your head with both hands at a point on the band which will give you the right amount of resistance.

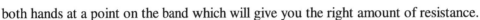

EXERCISES: 1. (a) Flex the L foot and turn the toes down into the floor. Use the L foot and the forehead as anchors for your balance.

(b) Bend the L knee slightly, if needed.

2. (a) Lift the R leg up behind you, keeping the leg straight, as high as it is comfortable.

(b) At the highest point, bend the R leg into an attitude position derriere (behind) and shorten the band.

(c) Cross the R leg (in attitude position) over the L leg.

(d) Try to touch the floor with the toes of the R foot on the other side of the L leg, reaching over as far as you can.

(e) As you return, initiate the movement by lifting the right foot and knee as high as possible.

(e) Rotate the hip back to center.

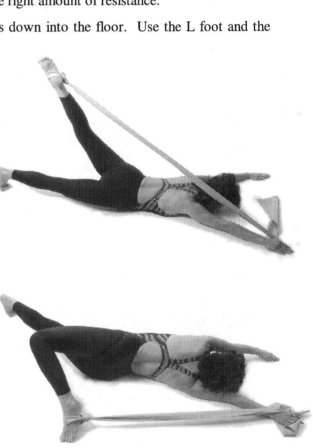

IV. DEEP ROTATION OF THE BACK II (ADVANCED)

POSITION: Lie on one side with both legs bent comfortably in front of the body; knee on top of knee, foot on top of foot. Straighten the arms on the floor directly in front of the shoulders, and have the elbows softened slightly.

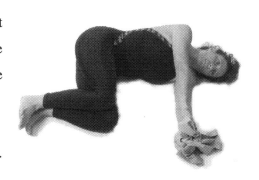

BAND: Hold the band a little wider apart than shoulder width.

EXERCISE: 1. Lengthen the upper arm forward, away from the body.

2. Lift the arm up toward the ceiling, creating a large an arc.

3 Keeping your arm at shoulder height, allow your head, eyes, neck and back to rotate with the upper arm.

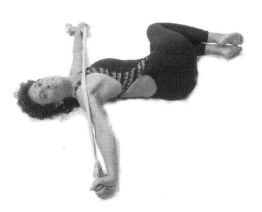

4. As you return to the beginning position, lengthen your arm away from your body and return, again, with the biggest arc you can create.

5. Work slowly, and exhale as you rotate you back in both directions.

V. PEARL NECKLACE

POSITION: Sit on your knees or on the edge of a chair.

Hold your arms overhead, slightly wider than shoulder width apart.

BAND: Hold the band overhead in both hands.

EXERCISES: NOTE: Throughout the exercises in this section,

think of each of the vertebrae in your spine as an individual pearl on

a necklace. As you curve your spine, each one is affected in progression.

1. (a) Lower your arms to shoulder height,

stretching the band behind your head.

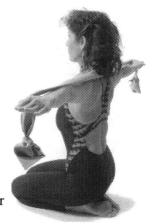

(b) Allow the head to roll downward, curving your tail/bone and tilting your

pelvis backward at the same time. This will lengthen your spine into a "C"

shape.

(c) Return by initiating the movement from the tail/bone.

VARIATION: Return by initiating the movement from the head and rolling

the spine up.

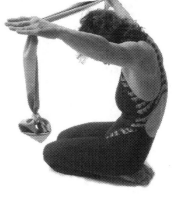

2. (a) As in number 1, tilt the pelvis backwards and roll the head forward

creating a "C" shape in your spine.

(b) Lower your arms (and the band) to shoulder height. While you are in that

position, rotate the torso to the L side without changing the relationship

between the arms and the body.

(c) Rotate back to the center and roll the spine back to the original position

one vertebra at a time.

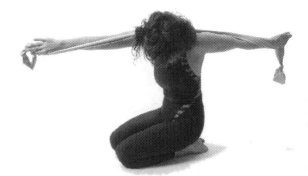

3. (a) Repeat number 2, except once you curve the spine into a "C" shape and rotate to the L side, you will lead with the L arm diagonally to the floor behind you into a high release and the R arm will go diagonally upward in front of your body.

 (b) Change the focus of your eyes and head upward to your R arm.

4. (a) Use your abdominal muscles to lift yourself with a hyper extended back into a sitting position.

(b) Face forward with your torso turned to the right side.

(c) Rotate the torso back to the center.

(d) Bring your arms overhead to the starting position.

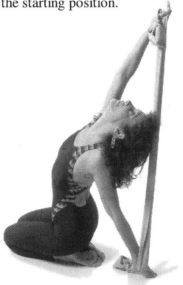

VI. HEAD AND NECK: THE GIRAFFE

POSITION : Sit comfortably on your knees, cross-legged, or on a chair, as long as your body remains in good alignment.

NOTE: (a) You will be using the band against the head to create resistance for stretching and strengthening the neck and head muscles.

(b) Please note the position of the head for each individual exercise.

EXERCISES:

1. (a) Spread the width of the band behind your head and over your ears.

(b) Pull the band forward in front of your face as you push your nose and chin

backwards. This will create a lengthening effect at the back of your neck.

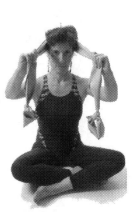

2. (a) Spread the width of the band across the forehead.

(b) Pull the back backward slightly to create tension.

(c) Push your entire head forward, not just the chin.

3. (a) Spread the band width over your L ear. Your L hand will hold one end of the

band in front of your face, and the R hand will hold the other end of

the band behind your head.

(b) Push the head to the L side, leading with your L ear.

(c) Repeat on the R side.

4. Side Stretch:

(a) Lower the R ear down towards the R shoulder, with the nose and chin facing forward.

(b) Spread the hand over your L ear from front to back (as in number 3).

(c) Slowly and gently pull the band down toward the R side. Sustain this position while

exerting very gentle pressure.

(d) Hold for one second, then release.

(e) Repeat on the other side.

5. Back of the Neck Stretch: Repeat number 4, except the band

will be wrapped along the back of the head. Your head will bend

forward as you gently apply pressure, as above.

VII. BASIC BARRE WORK

NOTE: (a) In each of the exercises in this section, you will need a ballet barre to use with the band. If you do not have access to a barre, other objects may be used instead: a doorknob, the edge of a **sturdy** piece of furniture, a strong towel rack, or a railing.

(b) Please note the body positions in the individual exercises.

BAND: Wrap the center of the band over the barre once or twice, as needed. The ends of the band will hang down.

EXERCISES:

1. (a) Attach the ends of the band to each ankle.

(b) Shift your body slightly back, away from the barre, in order to create tension in the band. Your feet are raised a little off the floor.

(c) Lower both legs toward the floor and return slowly.

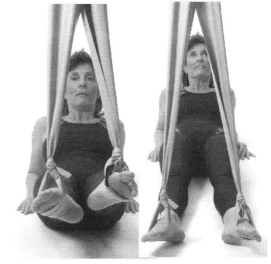

2. (a) Keep the band wrapped on your feet as you turn your body over to lie in a prone position (face down).

(b) Repeat number 1.

3. (a) Turn your body, so that your upper body is prone below the barre.

(b) Hold an end of the band in each hand and shift your body away from the barre to create tension in the lifted arms.

(c) Lower your arms to the floor and return slowly.

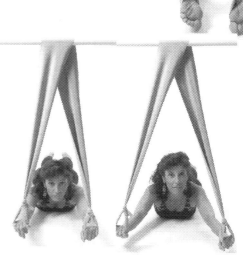

4. Repeat number 3 in a supine position.

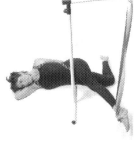

5. (a) Lie on your R side with lower leg bent and upper leg extended.

(b) Wrap both ends of the band on upper foot and the body is shifted

forward, so you are underneath the barre, in order to create tension in the band.

(c) Lower the upper leg to the floor.

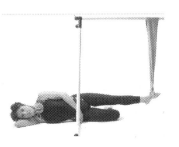
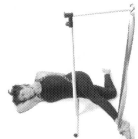

6. Repeat number 5, flexing the foot of the upper leg as you swing it gently backward and forward. Wrap one end of the band around the ankle, and the other end around the arch of the foot.

7. (a) Sit facing the barre with the ends of band on your ankles and your legs extended in front of you. Shift your body back slightly to create tension, but keep your heels on the floor.

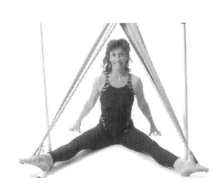

(b) Support your upper body with your fingers on the floor behind you and your elbows bent.

(c) Keep the abdominal muscles working against the back, which is straightened and lifted, not sunken back into the body. Shoulders are pressed down.

(d) Open your legs slowly to a wide second position; then close them again, being sure your heels stay on the floor.

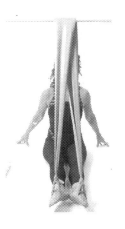

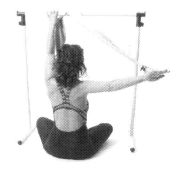

8. (a) Sit facing the barre, far enough away so you can extend both arms directly in front of you and touch the barre.

(b) Hold one end of the band with the R hand while you stabilize the other end on the barre with the L hand.

(c) Extend the R arm to the side and behind you on a diagonal, turning the upper body and head as you turn.

(d) Return slowly to the starting position.

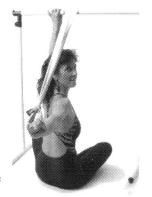

9. Repeat number 8, pressing your extended arm down to the floor after you rotate it behind you.

10. Sit in fourth position facing out from the barre, with the L leg in front of your body and the R leg behind you as far as possible. You will be positioned underneath the barre to create resistance.

(a) Lift the R foot off the floor. Both ends of the band are on your R foot.

(b) Lower the R foot down toward the ground by outwardly rotating the whole leg in the hip socket.

11. Sit in the same as in number 10.

(a) Extend the R leg directly behind you in an arabesque aligned behind the R side of your back.

(b) Return by releasing the knee into the floor and bending the lower leg back into the fourth position.

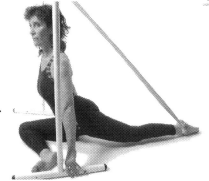

1

I came to America in 1982 with a strong idealism of what would create a fit body: adequate sleep, good nutrition, healthy relationships, comfort, natural fabrics and soft shoes. These were all in addition to basics: a good balance between flexibility and strength, aerobic fitness and endurance, and efficiency of movement and grace. But, always, I am also another human being. However, as I was adjusting to my new life here in America I watched television and spoke with people. The picture that I got of what Americans thought about their health was quite different. Gyms offer "lifetime memberships" where you could learn how to focus on isolating specific muscles and to strengthen them on machines, rather than learning how to integrate all of them in movement. I also saw how people repeatedly danced to rock and roll music in a way that is too hard on their joints in order to make their hearts race. Needless to say, I was surprised and a little disappointed.

2

People put a lot of thought and energy into making lives easier for themselves, disengaging themselves from things with "ease" in mind. For example, a mother is busy, and she cannot get anything done because the baby needs to be touched and carried all the time. The mother takes the child who can not sit, crawl, or walk yet, and puts him or her in a "walker," a rolling chair that keeps his back supported in a sitting position, so he can keep up with her. Do people think they can outsmart nature? Do we really believe that child will have a strong enough back to carry him through life when he is made to skip the necessary developmental stages on the floor? Could that be one of the reasons people miss days from work each year, to back problems?

3

At times, the days seem short, and the schedule is full of things that need to be done. One of the ways I cope with the stresses in my life is by doing a relaxation technique. It only takes five to ten minutes, but makes me feel rejuvenated once again. Lie down. Bring both knees up to your chest, legs about hip width apart. Let them drop down directly below you so the soles of your feet are on the floor and your knees are pointing up to the ceiling. If you feel pressure behind your lower back, you may put some support behind you, so the pelvis will rotate slightly backward. You may use a towel, pair of socks, small pillow, or even your own hand (open or in a fist). Close your eyes and focus inward. Visualize the space inside of your body entirely filled with sand or some kind of thick, slow-moving liquid, such as honey. Imagine little holes at certain places on the back side of your body--in the back of your skull, on each shoulder blade, on the pelvis (at each side of your spine), on the palms of your hands, and on the heels. Imagine the thick and heavy substance inside your body very slowly draining out of these holes and through the floor, just like grains of sand drain out of an hourglass. Once you find that you are "empty," you will be rested and ready to continue your busy day.

4

Through years of being a muscle therapist, I have grown to recognize movement in areas other than in physical bodies. Relationships also are constantly changing and dynamic. Traumatic emotional experiences can cause injuries to a person just as sure as the physical ones can. The similarity goes even further. If the trauma was severe enough, the person may also need the help of a different kind of therapist in order to heal. Most of the time, though, the disturbances that temporarily alter our balance are minor ones. Still, the way we choose to compensate for them may not be the most efficient way to handle the situation. In that case, it would be good to check our own emotional "alignment" every so often, to be certain that it can "support" us once again. I have found out for myself that one of my own personality traits is to push forward too strongly in my relationships. Sometimes, especially at the most important times, I have found that doing this did not serve me well at all. I am learning to let go a little, to stop forcing the issue as much, and I am pleasantly surprised to discover this change is creating a vacuum; a space for new movement and new rhythm to the relationship. For me, this new pattern I have chosen allows me to "move more easily" through some of my relationships.

5

I believe that as we grow up, we give up movement. We limit our possibilities. For example, look at our shoes. We wear shoes that will shape our feet, not shoes in the shape of our feet. It is the same thing with our clothing. In addition, some people will sit for hours in chairs and not move. They always sit at the same height and at the same angle. Are we designed for stationary positions or for activity? Are we really using the muscle possibility that is installed for us by nature?

6

How many people do you know who rub the back of their neck with their hands while talking to your or who would really enjoy a good neck massage? How many are in pain? There is a direct correlation between improper posture and the bio mechanics which cause a person's pain. In addition, dysfunctional movement patterns can cause physic pathological reflex arcs in the nervous system and can also increase the intra joint pressure in the facet joints of the vertebral column. This is why incorrect posture can give you a real pain in the neck!

7

In the summer of 1972, we were a group of teenagers who had just graduated from high school and who would soon be drafted into the Israeli army for two years of mandatory military service. We were willing to serve the country that we grew up in, but we also had mixed feelings. There was fear and doubt about the way the occupied territories were being dealt with. There were just a few days left before we would be drafted, so we decided to have a big party. We cut the boys' long hair (which was very symbolic in those days), and then we drove south to the Sinai desert seashore. There was a giant sand dune of dry, white sand which had all of its wrinkles smoothly ironed out by the wind. We climbed up one side to the top of it, looking out over the beach. Then, we shed our clothes and rolled all the way down the other side, leaving our own prints in the sand where it had once been perfectly smooth and empty. From the bottom of the sand dune, it was a short run to the water. What a sense of movement! What a sense of freedom!

PART 5

ESPECIALLY FOR

DANCERS

"UNIFIED AM I, QUITE UNDIVIDED, UNIFIED MY SOUL , UNIFIED MY SIGHT,
UNIFIED MY HEARING, UNIFIED MY BREATHING--BOTH IN AND OUT, UNIFIED IS MY
CONTINUOS BREATH, UNIFIED, QUITE UNDIVIDED AM I, THE WHOLE OF ME."
ATHAVA VEDA

MUSCLES FOR OUTWARD ROTATION OF THE HIP

1. Gluteus medius (in hip adduction)	E. Obturator internus
2. Gluteus maximus	F. Quadratus femoris
3. The six deep lateral rotator muscles	4. Iliopsoas (when thigh is flexed)
A. Piriformis	5. Sartorius (when thigh is flexed)
B. Gemellus superior	6. Biceps femoris
C. Gemelius	7. Adductor brevis (in hip adduction)
D. Obturator externus	8. Adductor magnus (in hip adduction)I.

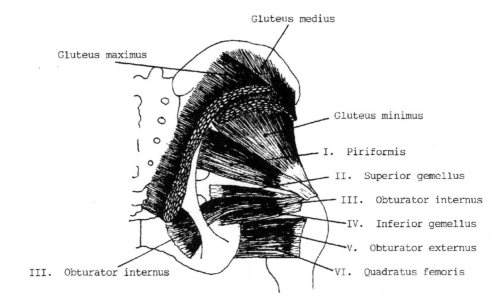

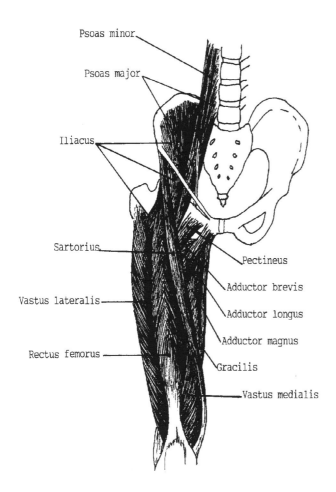

Psoas minor

Psoas major

Iliacus

Sartorius

Vastus lateralis

Rectus femorus

Pectineus

Adductor brevis

Adductor longus

Adductor magnus

Gracilis

Vastus medialis

I PREPARATION FOR ALLEGRO WORK

POSITION: Lie on your back with your legs at a 90° angle from the torso, with the soles of the feet flexed toward the ceiling. (An alternative position would be to sit in a parallel first position.)

BAND: Wrap the ends of the band on the feet, and hold the center of it in front of your chest.

EXERCISES: NOTE: numbers 1-5 are similar to the exercises under ANTI GRAVITY LEGWORK, but are included here again specifically as a preparation for jumps. When requested, do the exercises with **more energy and force**.

1. Turn your legs out, and then back to parallel several times.

2. (a) Bend your knees while your legs are in parallel, so your feet are on an imaginary line directly above your navel. Imagine another line that goes from the heels to the tail bone. Do not let the legs lean toward the face.

(b) Straighten the legs by lengthening them behind the knees. Push out with the heels.

3. (a) Turn your legs out, so your feet are in first position.

(b) Bend your knees into a demi-plie', opening the knees toward the sides.

(c) Straighten the legs by pushing the heels upward.

4. (a) Demi-plie' as in numbers 3. When both legs are bent, straighten the R leg into a tendu on a diagonal to the R side with both feet still flexed.

(b) Return to the diamond shape (demi-plie') and straighten the legs by pushing upward with the heels.

(c) Repeat to the other side.

5. CHANGEMENTS: (a) Turn out the legs and place one foot in front of the other foot, in a fifth position. (b) Open both legs a small distance to the side with the feet still flexed.

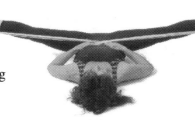

(c)Then, close to fifth position, changing which leg is in front.

6. Repeat number 5, opening your legs as wide as possible into second position on the "jumps".

7. (a) Keeping the legs in parallel, open them a little wider than hip width apart, in a parallel first position.

(b) Bend the legs into a demi-plie'.

(c) Push the leg forcefully up toward the ceiling.

8. Repeat number 7, except the legs are in a turned out first position with the heels together.

9. (a) Feet in a parallel first position with maximum flexion. Work just with the feet.

 (b) Point the feet with speed and force.

(c)Repeat this exercise with the feet in a turned out first position.

10. Repeat number 9 with feet in parallel second position and turned out second position.

11. Combine the force and the speed of the legs with the force and the speed of the feet. "Jump" up toward the ceiling, allowing your spine to lift off the floor. The feet are in each of the positions in numbers 9 and 10.

12. STAND. Attach the ends of the bands to each foot with the center of band over the shoulders and behind the head. You will be using the band resistance as you actually saute' in first and second positions--or any other jumping exercise that suits your needs.

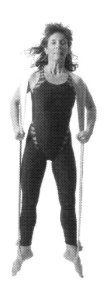
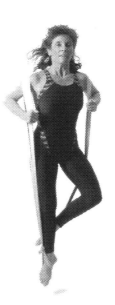
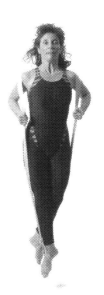

II. ADVANCED BARRE WORK

POSITION: Stand next to the barre, holding on to it with your L hand.

BAND: Attach both ends of the band to the R foot. Spread the center of the band across the L
shoulder.

EXERCISES: 1. PASSE'

(a) Stand in a turned out first position.

(b) Draw the R foot in a flexed position up the R leg as high as you can without
changing the level of your hipbones.

2. TENDU: (a) From first position, tendu the flexed R foot devant (forward) with the heel
going forward.

(b) Point the foot, then close the
foot again to first position by pulling
the toes back first.

(c) Do the tendu very slowly, spreading the toes
and going through demi-pointe each time.

(d) Repeat en croix.

3. Repeat number 2, except the R foot will degage'
instead of tendu.

4. Rond de jambe the R leg a' terre (on the floor) in
any combination you are   familiar
with, both en de dans (inward) and en de hors (outward); with the feet flexed
once, then pointed.

5. Repeat number 4, except the rond de jambe will be en l'air (in the air).

6. Use any frappe' combination you are familiar with in an en croix pattern.
You may either do your frappe's using the Cecchetti Method, where the foot will
be flexed at the ankle and pointed as it is extended, or the
Vaganova Method, where the foot is in sur le cou de pied
on the ankle before it is extended. You may also
choose to do a combination of both.

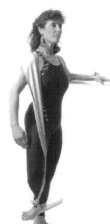

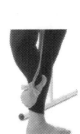

7. Develope' the R leg from first position through retire' passe' devant in any combination or at any height that your flexibility will permit. Repeat the combination en croix. You may use your R hand to increase the tension as your leg extends in each direction.

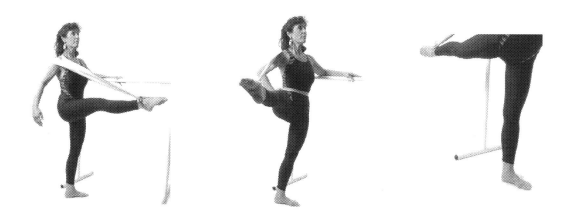

8. Grand battement the R leg en croix, making sure your body stays stable and adjusting the band tension if necessary.

9. (a) Attach each end of the band on the sole of each foot.

(b) Spread the center of the band is across your shoulders.

(c) Face the barre and hold the barre with both hands.

(d) Work on your jumps; small jumps in first and second positions, changements in fifth position, and even bigger jumps.

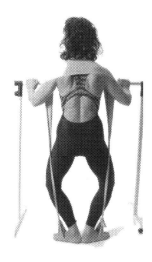
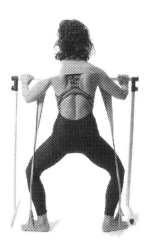

1

When a dancer comes to me before a performance with aches and pains, I usually will do just relaxation work with him or her, specifically avoiding any deep tissue work so as to not disturb his or her alignment. The alignment he or she is familiar with must remain his or her "comfort zone" until after show time--even if his or her present alignment which is causing stress on the body is the reason for his or her discomfort. Learning good alignment and correcting bad posture habits is a process that takes time and attention and is not something which can be "fixed" all at once.

2

Once we sustain an injury, it may become necessary to find an alternative way to handle movement. This way the stress can be redistributed through the body, rather than just on the injured part. I had a college athlete who came to see me because the swimming scholarship he had was about to be reevaluated. He had a severe elbow injury which held back his swimming progress. I looked at this swimming movement and observed he used primarily his arm and shoulder muscles, pushing through the pain, fighting his body to do what it was not ready to do yet. During our time together, I showed him how to initiate the swimming motion from his back muscles, which were strong and had not been injured. The arm would be able to carry the movement as a result, but the power would come from the back.

3

Occasionally, an injured student will come to me for a quick "miracle fix." With young adults (especially dancers), I can get muscles to respond faster and get time to let go of the tension sooner than with older people. However, even the youngest and most flexible bodies need more than instant "magic" to work with their injuries. It is important to treat the situation that caused the injury as well as the injury itself in order to prevent it happening again. You may even find that it is necessary to completely relearn a movement pattern in another way, so the same thing will not occur again. The injured area must be healed and strengthened. Look at your alignment in a functional way by asking yourself, "How can I move using the correct muscle to create balance and harmony?"

CHAPTER 3

CONCLUSION

As you have read and experimented with these exercises,.I hope you have been able to join me in the attitude and mind-set of awareness which I have tried to convey to you. I am sure that by now you have been able to recognize some of the benefits of using the Thera-Band® as you warm up and work out, such as the following:

A. providing the appropriate resistance in order to increase the strength and flexibility of the muscles;

B. allowing movement in three dimensions;

C. initiating movement from the pelvis;

D. integrating different body parts to achieve harmonious and athletic movement;

E. getting in touch with the abilities of the spine--extension, flexion, and rotation--and recognizing the relationship between the head and the tail/bone;

F. providing support and balance, in some exercises;

G. allowing the full range of movement (for example, using the complete range capabilities of the hip when turning).

H. providing a reference for posture and alignment which will reflect on your everyday activities; and finally,

I. providing the tactile sensation on the skin, thus provoking greater awareness. Some elements of movement were not explored in this book (for example, using the band as a help for weight transference). I hope you will continue to work with the Thera-Band® , using your own knowledge and creativity to develop other exercises which are specifically suited to meeting the needs of your own individual body.

SUGGESTED READING

Alexander, E Matthias. *The Alexander Technique: The Essential Writings of F. Matthias Alexander.* Selected and introduced by Edward Maisel. London: Thames and Hudson, 1990.

~. *The Use of the Self.* New York: E. P. Dutton & Co., 1932. Reprint. Long Beach, CA: Centerline Press, 1984.

Alexander, Gerda. Eutony: *The Holistic Discovery of the Total Person.* New York: Felix Morrow, 1985

Alter, Michael J. *Science of Stretching.* Champaign, IL: Human Kinetics Books, 1988.

---~-. Sport Stretch. Champaign, IL: Leisure Press, 1990.

Brooks, Charles V.W. *Sensory Awareness: The Rediscovery of Experiencing Through Workshops With Charlotre Selver.* New York: Viking Press, 1974. Reprint. New York: Felix Morrow, 1986.

Chmelar, Robin D. and Sally S. Fitt. *Dancing at Your Peak: Diet: A Complete Guide To Nutrition and Weight Control.* Pennington, NJ: Princeton Book Company, 1990.

Clarkson, Priscilla M. and Margaret Skrinar, eds. *Science of Dance training.* Champaign, 1L: Human Kinetics Books, 1988.

Clarkson, Priscilla, Oded Bar-Or, and David R. Lamb. *Exercise and the Female: A Life Span Approach.* Perspectives in Exercise Science and Sports Medicine, vol. 9. Carmel, 1N: Cooper Publishing Group, 1996.

Cohen, Bonnie Bainbridge. *"The Action in Perceiving,"* Contact Quarterly, 12, no. 3 (Fall 1987): 22-26.

~. *"The Dancer's Warm-up through Body-Mind Centering."* Contact Quarterly, 13, no. 3 (Fall 1988): 28-29.

~. *"Perceiving in Action,"* Contact Quarterly, 9, no. 2 (Spring/Summer 1984). 24-39.

~. *"Relationship of the Concept of Proximal and Distal lnitiation to Muscle Structure and Function."* Amherst, MA: The School for Body/Mind Centering, 1977.

~. *Sensing, Feeling, and Action: The Experiential Anatomy of Body-Mind Centering*: The Collected Articles from Contact Quarterly Dance Journal, 19801- 1992. Northampton, MA: Contact Editions, 1993.

Dowd, Irene. *Taking Root to Fly: Ten Articles on Functional Anatomy.* New York: Contact Collaborations, Inc., 1981. 3rd rev. ed. New York: lrene Dowd, 1995.

Feldenkrais, Moshe. Awareness Through Movement: Health Exercises for Personal Growth. New York: Harper & Row, Publishers, Inc., 1972. Reprint. New York: Har Per Collins, 1990.

~. *The Elusive Obvious.* Cupertino, CA: Meta Publications, 1981.

-- *The Potent Self: A Guide to Spontaneity.* New York: Harper & Row, Publishers, Inc., 1985. Reprint. San Francisco: Harper San Francisco, 1992.

Firt,,Salley ,Sevey. *Dance Kinesiology 2nd edition.* New York: Schirmer Books, 1996.

Friden, J. *"Changes in Human Skeletal Muscle Induced by long term Eccentric Exercise."* Cell Tissue Research, 236, no. 2 (1984): 365-372,

Friden, J., Sjostrom, M., and B. Ekblom. Experimentia 37, no. 5 (1981): 506-507.

Grant, Gail. *Technical Manual and Dictionary of Classical Ballet,* third revised edition New York: Dover Publications, Inc., 1982.

Hoppenfeld, Stanley and Richard Hutton. *Physical Examination of the Spine and Extremities.* Norwalk, CT: Appelton-Century-Crofts, 1976.Hygienic Corporation.

Tera-Band® System of Progressive Resistance: Instruction Manual, vol.3.OH: The Hygienic Corporation, 1992.

Juhan, Dean. *Job's Body: A Handbook for Bodywork.* Barrington, New York: Station Hill Press/Barrytown, 1987 Expended edition. Barrington, NY: Berrytown. Ltd, 1998.

Kapit, Wynn and Lawrencc M. Elson. *The Anatomy Coloring Book.* New York: Harper Collins Publishers, Inc., 1977 Second edition. New York: Addison Wesley Publishing Company: 1993.

Kedall Florence Peterson and Elizabeth Kendall McCreary. *Muscles: Testing and Function,* Fourth edition, Baltimore: Iippincott, Williams & Wilkins, 1993.

Kirseitin, Lincoln and Muriel Stuart. *The Classical Ballet: Basic Technique and Terminology.* New York: Alfred A. Knopf, lnc., 1952. Reprint, Gainsville: University Press of Florida, 1998.

Lao Tzu. *Tao Te Ching.* Translated by Victor H. Mair. New York: Quality Paperback Book Club, 1990.

Linden, Paul. *Compute in comfort.* Saddle River, NJ: Prentice-Hall, Inc., 1995.

-- *"Being in Movement: Intention as a Somatic Meditation.* Somatics, (Autumn/ Winter 1988-89): 54-59

McMinn, R.M.H. and R. T.Hutchings. *A Color Atlas of Human Anatomy.* London: Wolfe Medical Publications Ltd., 1977.

Mariechild, Diane. *The Inner Dance Freedom,* CA Crossing Press, 1987.

Marks, S. C., R. M. McMinn, Peter H. Abrahams, and Halph T, Hutchings. McMinn's *Color Atlas of Human Anatomy,* Fourth Edition. London: Mosby-Year Book, 1998.

McAtee. Robert E. *Facilitated Stretching.* Colorado Springs, CO: Human Kinetics Publishers, 1993.

Minton, Sandra Cerny. *Body and Self: Partners in Movement.* Champaign, IL: Human Kinetics Publishers 1989.

Morris, Christofer M. *The Complete Guide to Stretching.* London: A. &C. Black, Ltd., 1999.

Nelson Lisa, and Nancy Stark Smith. *"Interview with Bonnie Bainbridge Cohen."* Contact Quarterly 5,no.2(Winter 1980) :20-28.

Newham, D. J., G. McPhail, K. R. Mills, &, R. H. T. Edwards. *"Ultra Structural Changes after Concentric and Eccentric Contrasction of Human Muscle."* Journal of the Neuro logical Sciences, 61, no.1 (1983): 109-122.

Olsen, Andrea, in collaboration with Caryn McHose. Body Stories: A Guide to Experimental Anatomy. Barrytown, NY: Station Hill Press, Inc., 1991. Expanded edition. Barrytown, NY: Station Hill Ltd., 1999.

Rolf, Ida, PhD, Rolfing: The Integration of Human Structure. New York: Harper & Row Publishers, 1977.

Saltonstall, Ellen. Kinetic Awareness: Discovering Your Body mind. New York: Kinetic Awareness Center, 1988.

School for Body/Mind Centering. Ontogenetic and Phylogenetic Deuelopmental Pninci-ples, revised edition. Amherst, MA: School for Body/Mind Centering, 1977.

Organs: Lungs, Heart, Kidneys, Bladder, Gonads, revised edition. Amherst, MA: School for Body/Mind Centering, 1977.

Selim, Robert D. *Muscles: The Magic of Motion: The Human Body. Human Body Series.* D.C.:U.U.S. News & World Report, Inc., 1982.

Smith, Fritz Frederick. *lnner Bridges: A Guide to Energy Movement and Body Structure.* Atlanta, GA: Humanics Publishing Group, 1986.

Smith, Nancy Stark. "Living Anatomy of Vision: interview With Bonnie Bainbridge Cohen." Contact Quarterly, 6: no. 1 (winter 1981): 5-9.

Spector-Flock, Noa. *"The Power of Stretching with a Band."* Unpublished article, 2001.

Syer, John and Christopher Connolly. *Sporting Body, Sporting Mind: An Athlete's Guide to Mental Training.* Englewood, NJ: Prentice-Hall, Inc., 1989.

Thomason, Eivind and Rachel-Anne Rist. *Anatomy and Kinesiology for Ballet Teachers.* London: Dance Books, 1996

Thompson, Clem W. *Manual of Structural Kinesiology,* 11 th edition. St. Louis, MO: Times Mirror/Mosby College Publishing, 1989.

Thoreau, Henry David. *Walden and Other Writings.* New York: Barnes and Noble, 1993.

Tavell, Janet G. and David G. Simons. *Myofascial pain and Dysfunction: The Trigger Point Manual.* 2 vols. Second Edition. Baltimore: Lippincott, Williams & Wilkins, 1998.

Watkins, Andrea and priscilla M. Clarkson. *Dancing Longer, Dancing Stronger: A Dan-cer's Guide to Improving Technique and Preventing Injury.* Pennington Book Company, 1990.

1. ABDUCTORS: any muscle group that will bring a particular body part away from the mid-line of the body (i.e., raising the arm out to the side).

2. ADDUCTORS: any muscle group that will bring a particular body part closer to the body's mid-line (i.e., when sitting on a chair and crossing one leg over the other, the inner thigh muscle will adduct the leg over the other leg.)

3. ANTERIOR: the front side of the body or specific body part.

4. CIRCUMDUCTION: the moving of a bone in a circular pattern from a single axis, creating a cone shape in space.

5. CONCENTRIC: when the distance between muscle ends becomes shorter in a contraction.

6. CONTRACTION: the building of tension in a muscle or muscle group.

7. DEPRESSION: the downward motion of a body part, or the returning movement from elevation.

8. DORSAL: the upper side of a body part.

9. ECCENTRIC: when muscle fibers become more extended and the distance between the two muscle ends is greater in a contraction.

10. ELEVATION: the upward motion of a body part.

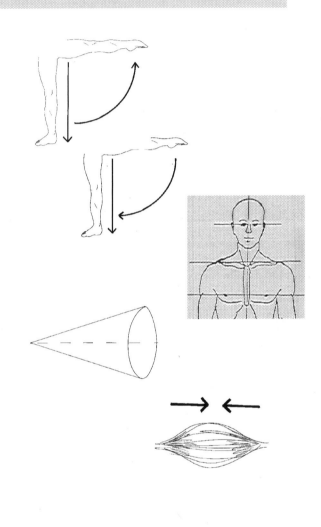

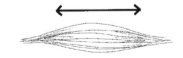

11. EVERSION: the outward rotation of the foot from the mid-line of the body.

12. EXTENSION: straightening; moving bones apart to make the angle between them wider.

13. FIXATION: the stabilizing or fixating one area of the body while another area moves freely.

14. FLEXED FOOT: the bringing of the dorsal side of the foot and all toes toward the face.

15. FLEXION: the bending of a joint where the angle between two bones becomes smaller.

16. FRONTAL PLANE: a division of the body from one side to the other which creates separate back and front regions.

17. HORIZONTAL EXTENSION (ABDUCTION): the movement of a body part horizontally from the front of the body to the side.

18. HORIZONTAL FLEXION (ADDUCTION): movement of a body part horizontally from the side of the body to the front.

19. HORIZONTAL PLANE: a division of the body at the waistline which creates an upper region and a lower region of the body.

20. HYPEREXTENSION: when a joint (especially the knee and elbow joints) which is designed to flex in only one direction is

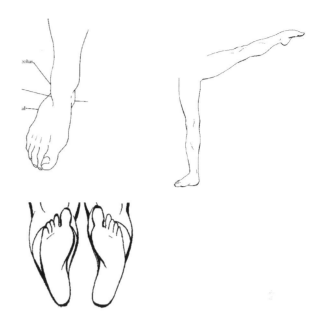

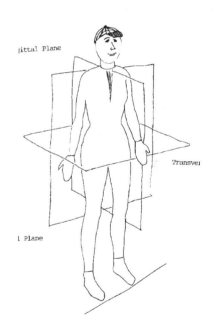

straightened to a locked position, sometimes to the point that it begins to flex in the opposite direction.

21. INVERSION: the turning of the foot, for example, so the sole is facing toward the mid-line of the body.

22. ISCHIAL TUBEROSITY: one of the "sitting bones"; the lowest of the three protruding bones of the pelvis (the others being the iliac crest and the pubis).

23. LATERAL: the outer side or aspect of the body or a body part.

24. LUMBAR REGION: the five vertebrae located between the mid-back and the top of the hip at the waistline.

25. MEDIAL: the inner aspect of the body or body part closest to the midline of the body.

26. METATARSAL: the section of the foot between the toes and the arch.

27. PLANTAR: the lower side or aspect of the body part; for example, the sole of the foot.

28. POINTED FOOT: the plantar flexion of the foot.

29. POSTERIOR: the back side of the body.

30. PRONE POSITION: lying on your abdominal muscles, face down.

31. ROTATION: the moving of a bone along its own axis.

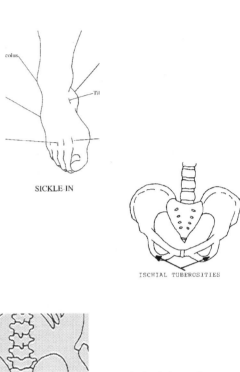

SICKLE IN

ISCHIAL TUBEROSITIES

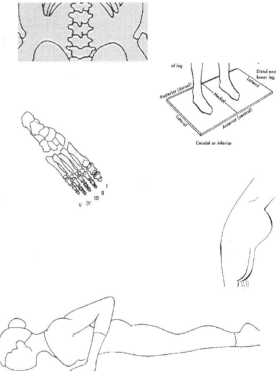

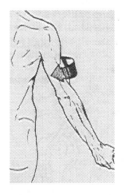

32. SACRUM: the flat, triangular-shaped bone located on the posterior aspect of the pelvis, at the end of the lumbar area and between the two iliac crests (hipbones).

33. SAGITTAL PLANE: a division at the center of the body which creates symmetrical right and left sides.

34. SCAPULA: the shoulder blade.

35. SICKLED FOOT: the disruption of good foot alignment caused by turning the toes inward, as if you were looking at the sole of your foot.

36. SUPINE POSITION: lying on your back, face upward.

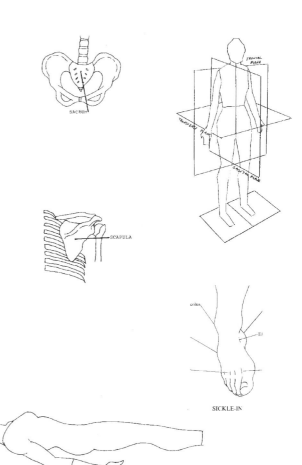

APPENDIX B: BALLET TERMS
Russian Style

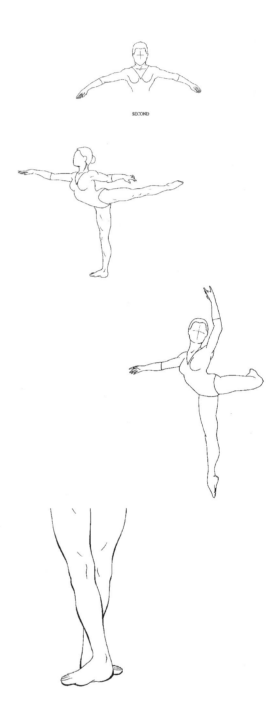

SECOND

1. A' LA SECOND: a positioning of the arms or the legs directly to the side of the body, as if in a second position.

2. ARABESQUE: a body position in which you are supported on one leg, which may be bent or straight. The other leg is extended directly behind you, usually at 90 from the standing leg. The arms have several positions which can be used to create a long line from the toes to the fingers. Both shoulders are equal, as well as both hips, and both are at right angles to the line of direction.

3. ATTITUDE: a body position in which you are standing on one leg with the other leg lifted directly front (devant), side (a' la second), or behind (derriere). The knee is bent at a 90° angle from thigh to lower leg.

4. CHANGEMENT: a jump straight up in the air during which the feet switch from a fifth position with one foot in front to land in a fifth position with the other foot in front.

5. DERRIÈRE: a stationary position or movement that is done directly behind the body.

6. DEVANT: a stationary position or movement done directly to the front of the body.

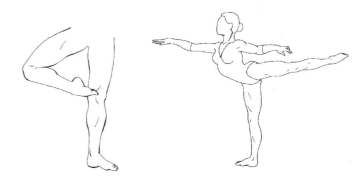

7. DEVELOPPÉ: a stationary movement that is done while standing on one leg. The other thigh is lifted, but the toes of the lifting leg touch the standing leg as it is drawn up. As soon as the thigh reaches maximum height, it is held there while the lower leg leaves the standing leg and is fully extended to a straightened position in the air.

8. EN CROIX: literally, "in the shape of a cross"; working in all directions--front, side, back, and side of the body again.

9. PLIÉ: a bend of the knees while standing. It can be DEMI-PLIÉ (half bend), in which the torso goes as low as possible when the knees bend, the heels not lifting off the floor, or else it can be GRANDE PLIÉ (large bend), a deep bend of the knees in which the heels do come off the floor (except in second position).

10. RELEVÉ (HALF TOE): standing on one or both feet, lift the heels off the floor so your weight is on the balls of your feet.

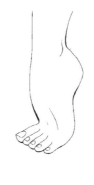

11. RETIRÉ: literally "withdrawn"; a position in which the thigh is lifted.

12. ROND DE JAMBE: a circular movement of the leg. It can be done with the toes remaining on the floor (a terre) or with the leg lifted in the air (en l'air), and the circle can be outward (en de hors) or inward (en de dans).

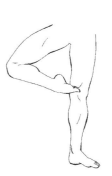

13. SAUTE': a jump straight up in the air. The position is the same before the jump and after it; it does not change in the air.

14. SUR LE COU DE PIED: a stationary position with the sole of one foot wrapped around the ankle of the standing foot, so that the heel can be seen from the front and the toes are behind the Achilles's tendon of the standing foot.

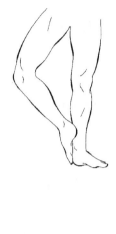

15. TENDU: a stationary movement standing on one leg. The other foot slides out in a particular direction (the knee is straight) with the toes remaining on the floor.

16. TURN-OUT: the outward rotation of the legs in the hip sockets, very important and basic to all ballet movements and positions.

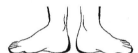

APPENDIX C : POSITIONS OF THE FEET, LEGS, BODY, AND ARMS

1. ALL FOURS POSITION: body weight is on the hands and knees, with the thighs and the arms at a 90 degree angle from the torso.

2. BALLET POSITIONS OF THE ARMS: Russian Style

A. FIRST POSITION: arms are held out in front of the body in a circular position, so the hands are at about the height of your navel, elbows are slightly bent and facing outward, tips of the fingers almost touching.

B. SECOND POSITION: arms are in the same shape as first position, except they are held out to each side of the body.

C. THIRD POSITION: arms are in the same shape as first position, except both arms are lifted so the hands are above the head.

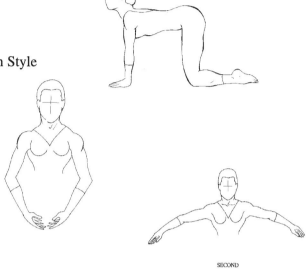

SECOND

3. BALLET POSITIONS OF THE FEET:

A. FIRST POSITION: heels are together, legs are turned out at the hip socket so the toes and knees point out from each other on a diagonal.

B. SECOND POSITION: same as first position, except feet are about hip width apart.

C. THIRD POSITION: rarely used; similar to first position, except the heel of one foot is touching the instep of the other foot.

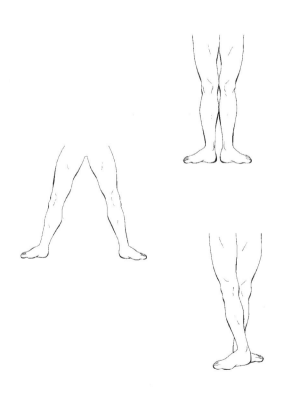

D. FOURTH POSITION: same as fifth position, below, except one foot is positioned a little ways directly in front of the other one.

E. FIFTH POSITION: legs are rotated outward at the hip; one foot is in front of the other, so that the lateral aspect of the heel of the front foot is touching the big toe of the back foot. (Ideally, the little toe of the front foot is touching the medial aspect of the heel of the back foot as well.)

4. SITTING FOURTH POSITION: sitting on the floor, one leg is bent in a 90 degree angle in front of the body, turned outward, and the other leg is bent in a 90 degree angle behind the body, turned inward; this creates an open square shape with the legs.

5. SITTING PARALLEL FIRST POSITION: sitting on the floor, legs are directly forward, the legs are in front of the hips, knees straight.

6. SITTING WIDE SECOND POSITION: straddle split; legs are open to each side of the body as you are seated on the ground, knees straightened and directed toward the ceiling.

7. STANDING PARALLEL FIRST POSITION: feet are parallel to each other, a few inches apart.

8. STANDING PARALLEL SECOND POSITION: feet are parallel to each other, about hip width apart.

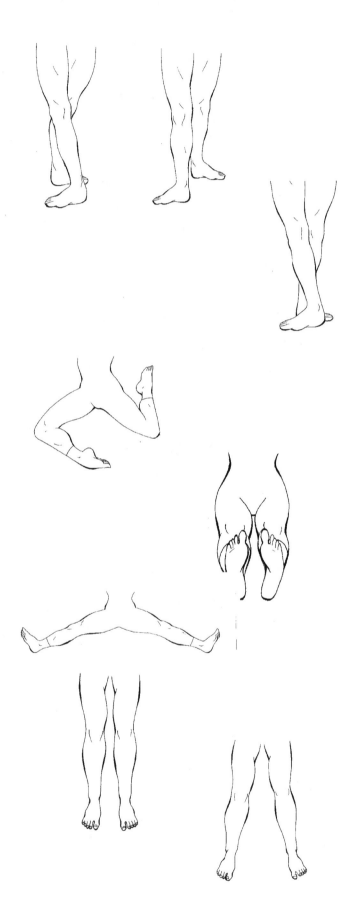

APPENDIX D: THREE-PART WHOLE BODY PROGRAM (SAMPLE)

I. FIRST DAY

I. ALTERNATING DAY

I. FIRST DAY	I. ALTERNATING DAY
1. Abdominal: The Ice Cream Scooper	1. Abdominal: The Ice Cream Scooper
2. Abdominal: Rotation	2. Abdominal: Rotation
3. Iliopsoas Stretch	3. Iliopsoas Stretch
4. Leg "Metic-ha" (Stretch)	4. Leg "Metic-ha" (Stretch)
5. Spinal Chain	5. Spinal Chain
6. Antigravity Legwork (#s 1-4)	6. Arms: The Traffic Director (#s 1-6)
7. Lying On One Side (#s 1-10)	7. Chest Press
8. The Hinge	8. "Tza-eef" (The Shawl)
9. The Little Mermaid Tail	9. Crescent Bend
10. The Pendulum	10. "Tzedadeem" (Laterals
11. The Body Builder (# 1 only)	11. The Body Builder
12. Prone: The Archer's Bow	12. Prone: The Archer's Bow (# 2 only)
13. Deep Rotation of the Back I	13. Pearl NecklaceII.
14. Antigravity Footwork	
15. Pearl NecklaceI.	

II FIRST DAY   II ALTERNATING DAY

1. Abdominal: The Ice Cream Scooper	1. Abdominal: The Ice Cream Scooper
2. Abdominal: Rotation	2. Abdominal: Rotation
3. Abdominal: Combination	3. Abdominal: Combination
4. Iliopsoas Stretch	4. Iliopsoas Stretch
5. Spinal Chain	5. Spinal Chain
6. Antigravity Legwork	6. Arms: The Traffic Director (# 1 and 7-10)
7. "Ameeda" (Standing) Legwork (#s 1-7)	7. Biceps
8. Lying On One Side (#s 1-10)	8. Triceps
9. Posterior: The Jungle Cat (#s 1-3 and 6-8)	9. Crescent Bend
10. Leg Adductors	10. Hands of the Clock
11. "Ain-soff" (Infinity Symbol:)	11. The Body Builder
12. The Body Builder (all)	12. Prone: The Archer's Bow (# 2 only)
13. Prone: The Archer's Bow	13. Pearl Necklace III.
14. Deep Rotation of the Back	

III.

1. Abdominal: The Ice Cream Scooper	8. "Tza-eef" (The Shawl)
2. Abdominal: Rotation	9. Shawl Variation
3. Abdominal: Combination	10. Crescent Bend
4. Iliopsoas Stretch	11. Crescent Twist
5. Spinal Chain	12. "Tzedadeem" (Laterals)
6. Arms: The Traffic Director (#s 1, 3-5, and 7)	13. Advanced "Tzedadeem" (Laterals)
7. Chest Press	12. The Body Builder (All)
	13. Pearl Necklace

APPENDIX E: PROGRAM FOR DANCE CONDITIONING

(SAMPLE)   FIRST DAY   ALTERNATING DAY

FIRST DAY	ALTERNATING DAY
1. Abdominal: The Ice Cream Scooper	1. Abdominals: The Ice Cream Scooper
2. Abdominals: Rotation	2. Abdominals: Rotation
3. Abdominals: Combination	3. Abdominals: Combination
4. Iliopsoas Stretch	4. Iliopsoas Stretch
5. Spinal Chain	5. Spinal Chain
6. Leg "Metic-ha" (Stretch)	6. Arms: The Traffic Director (#s 1-4)
7. Antigravity Legwork	7. "Tza-eef" (The Shawl)
8. Advanced Anti-Gravity Legwork	8. Chest Press
9. "Ameeda" (Standing) Legwork (for plie', balance, extension)	9. Crescent Bend
10. Lying On One Side (#s 1-10; for passe' retire'and extension)	10. Half-moon Twist
11. The Hinge	11. "Tzedadeem" (Laterals)
12. Posterior: The Jungle Cat (#s 4, 5, 7, 8)	12. Advanced "Tzedadeem" (Laterals)
13. The Little Mermaid Tail	13. The Body Builder
14. The Pendulum (#s 1-3)	14. Prone: The Archer's Bow
15. Leg Adductors	15. Deep Rotation of the Back I
16. Antigravity Footwork	16. Deep Rotation of the Back II
17. Calf and Foot: Revving the Accelerator	17. Pearl Necklace
18. The Body Builder	
19. Prone: The Archer's Bow	
20. Deep Rotation of the Back I	
21. Deep Rotation of the Back II	
22. Pearl Necklace	

APPENDIX F: PROGRAM FOR SWIM CONDITIONING

(SAMPLE) FIRST DAY	ALTERNATING DAY
1. Abdominals: The Ice Cream Scooper	1. Abdominals: The Ice Cream Scooper
2. Abdominals: Rotation	2. Abdominals: Rotation
3. Abdominals: Combination (for the warm-up of the back)	3. Abdominals: Combination
4. Iliopsoas Stretch	4. Iliopsoas Stretch
5. Lying On One Side (#s 1 and 2 to learn hip separation; #3 to strengthen the tensor fascia lata).	5. Lying On One Side (#s 1, 2, and 3)
6. The Hinge	6. The Hinge
7. The Little Mermaid Tail (for posterior hip muscle)	7. "Ain-soff" (Infinity Symbol:∞)
8. Leg Adductors (for breast-stroke)	8. Arms: The Traffic Director (#s 1-8)
9. "Ain-soff" (Infinity Symbol: ∞) (for overall coordination of leg and hip)	9. Chest Press
10. Prone: The Archer's Bow	10. Biceps
11. Deep Rotation of the Back I	11. Triceps
12. Deep Rotation of the Back II	12. "Tza-eef" (The Shawl)
13. Antigravity Footwork	13. Crescent Bend (for the side rib muscles)
14. Calf And Foot: Revving the Accelerator	14. The Body Builder

To order a band and three videos please contact

Noa Spector- Flock

7867 Country Club RD N.

St. Pete FL, 33710

U.S.A.

Tel: 1-727-345-2570

Email: noanik8@att.net

Printed in the United States
By Bookmasters